Gastroenterology

Editor

SEYMOUR KATZ

CLINICS IN
GERIATRIC MEDICINE

www.geriatric.theclinics.com

February 2014 • Volume 30 • Number 1

ELSEVIER

1600 John F. Kennedy Boulevard • Suite 1800 • Philadelphia, Pennsylvania, 19103-2899

http://www.theclinics.com

CLINICS IN GERIATRIC MEDICINE Volume 30, Number 1
February 2014 ISSN 0749–0690, ISBN-13: 978-0-323-28082-2

Editor: Jessica McCool
Developmental Editor: Yonah Korngold

Clinics in Geriatric Medicine (ISSN 0749-0690) is published quarterly by Elsevier Inc., 360 Park Avenue South, New York, NY 10010-1710. Months of issue are February, May, August, and November. Business and Editorial Offices: 1600 John F. Kennedy Blvd., Suite 1800, Philadelphia, PA 191023-2899. Periodicals postage paid at New York, NY, and additional mailing offices. Subscription prices are $280.00 per year (US individuals), $498.00 per year (US institutions), $145.00 per year (US student/resident), $370.00 per year (Canadian individuals), $632.00 per year (Canadian institutions), $195.00 per year (Canadian student/resident), $390.00 per year (foreign individuals), $632.00 per year (foreign institutions), and $195.00 per year (foreign student/resident). Foreign air speed delivery is included in all *Clinics* subscription prices. All prices are subject to change without notice. POSTMASTER: Send address changes to *Clinics in Geriatric Medicine*, Elsevier Health Sciences Division, Subscription Customer Service, 3251 Riverport Lane, Maryland Heights, MO 63043. Telephone: 1-800-654-2452 (U.S. and Canada); 314-447-8871 (outside U.S. and Canada). Fax: 314-447-8029. E-mail: journalscustomerservice-usa@elsevier.com (for print support) or journalsonlinesupport-usa@elsevier.com (for online support).

Reprints. For copies of 100 or more, of articles in this publication, please contact the Commercial Reprints Department, Elsevier Inc., 360 Park Avenue South, New York, New York 10010-1710. Tel.: 212-633-3874; Fax: 212-633-3820, E-mail: reprints@elsevier.com.

Clinics in Geriatric Medicine is covered in *MEDLINE/PubMed (Index Medicus)*, *EMBASE/Excerpta Medica, Current Contents/Clinical Medicine (CC/CM)*, and the *Cumulative Index to Nursing & Allied Health Literature*.

Printed and bound by CPI Group (UK) Ltd, Croydon, CR0 4YY

Transferred to digital print 2012

Contributors

EDITOR

SEYMOUR KATZ, MD, FACP, MACG
Clinical Professor of Medicine, New York University School of Medicine, New York; North Shore University Hospital, Long Island Jewish Hospital System, Manhasset; St. Francis Hospital, Roslyn, New York

AUTHORS

SADRA AZIZI, MD
Resident Physician, Albany Medical Center, Albany, New York

DAVID E. BERNSTEIN, MD, FACG, AGAF, FACP
Chief, Division of Hepatology and Center for Liver Disease; Professor of Medicine, Hofstra North Shore Long Island Jewish School of Medicine, North Shore Long Island Jewish Health System, Manhasset, New York

RICHARD CARMONA, BA
New York University School of Medicine, New York, New York

SHAWN CHAUDHARY, MD
Gastroenterology Fellow, Division of Gastroenterology, Albany Medical Center, Albany, New York

VANESSA C. COSTILLA, MD
Resident, Department of Internal Medicine, Mayo Clinic in Arizona, Scottsdale, Arizona

LUKEJOHN W. DAY, MD
Division of Gastroenterology, Department of Medicine, San Francisco General Hospital and Trauma Center, San Francisco, California

ANUPAMA T. DUDDEMPUDI, MD
Division of Hepatology, North Shore University Hospital; Assistant Professor of Medicine, Hofstra North Shore Long Island Jewish School of Medicine, Manhasset, New York

AMY E. FOXX-ORENSTEIN, DO, FACG, FACP
Associate Professor of Medicine, Division of Gastroenterology, Mayo Clinic in Arizona, Scottsdale, Arizona

JESSE GREEN, MD
Professor of Medicine, Division of Gastroenterology, Albany Medical Center, Albany, New York

SETH GROSS, MD
Division of Gastroenterology, Langone Medical Center, New York University, New York, New York

CHRISTINA Y. HA, MD
Clinical Assistant Professor, Division of Digestive Diseases, Center for Inflammatory Bowel Diseases, The David Geffen School of Medicine at the University of California, Los Angeles, Los Angeles, California

HENRY A. HORTON, MD
Division of Gastroenterology, Department of Medicine, Cedars-Sinai Medical Center, Los Angeles, California

PHILIP O. KATZ, MD
Chairman, Division of Gastroenterology, Albert Einstein Medical Center; Clinical Professor of Medicine, Thomas Jefferson University, Philadelphia, Pennsylvania

SEYMOUR KATZ, MD, FACP, MACG
Clinical Professor of Medicine, New York University School of Medicine, New York; North Shore University Hospital, Long Island Jewish Hospital System, Manhasset; St. Francis Hospital, Roslyn, New York

JONATHAN M. KELLER, MD
Internal Medicine Resident, Department of Medicine, University of Washington School of Medicine, Seattle, Washington

ABRAHAM KHAN, MD
Clinical Instructor of Medicine, Division of Gastroenterology, Department of Medicine, Center for Esophageal Disease, New York University School of Medicine, New York, New York

HAYOON KIM, MD
Division of Gastroenterology, Department of Medicine, Cedars-Sinai Medical Center, Los Angeles, California

GIL Y. MELMED, MD, MS
Associate Clinical Professor of Medicine, Division of Gastroenterology, Department of Medicine, Cedars-Sinai Medical Center, Los Angeles, California

DARRELL S. PARDI, MD, MS
Professor of Medicine, Vice Chair, Division of Gastroenterology and Hepatology, Inflammatory Bowel Disease Clinic, Mayo Clinic College of Medicine, Rochester, Minnesota

SATISH S.C. RAO, MD, PhD, FRCP (LON)
Professor of Medicine, Division of Gastroenterology and Hepatology, Medical College of Georgia, Georgia Regents University, Augusta, Georgia

FARID RAZAVI, MD
Division of Gastroenterology, Langone Medical Center, New York University, New York, New York

FELICE H. SCHNOLL-SUSSMAN, MD
Associate Professor of Clinical Medicine, Division of Gastroenterology and Hepatology, Department of Medicine, Weill Cornell Medical College, New York, New York

MANDEEP SINGH, MD
Gastroenterology Fellow, Division of Gastroenterology, Albany Medical Center, Albany, New York

AMIR SOUMEKH, MD
Clinical Fellow, Division of Gastroenterology and Hepatology, Department of Medicine, Weill Cornell Medical College, New York, New York

CHRISTINA M. SURAWICZ, MD
Professor of Medicine, Division of Gastroenterology, Department of Medicine, University of Washington School of Medicine, Seattle, Washington

MORRIS TRAUBE, MD, JD
Professor of Medicine, Division of Gastroenterology, Department of Medicine; Director, Center for Esophageal Disease, New York University School of Medicine, New York, New York

FERNANDO VELAYOS, MD, MPH
Division of Gastroenterology, Department of Medicine, University of California, San Francisco, San Francisco, California

SIEGFRIED W.B. YU, MD, FACP
Gastroenterology Fellow, Division of Gastroenterology and Hepatology, Medical College of Georgia, Georgia Regents University, Augusta, Georgia

Contents

Most oropharyngeal dysphagia are of neurologic origin, and management is coordinated with a clinical swallow specialist in conjunction with an ear, nose, and throat (ENT) physician if warning signs imply malignancy. Several structural and functional esophageal disorders can cause dysphagia. If a patient has likely esophageal dysphagia, a video barium esophagram is a good initial test, and referral to a gastroenterologist is generally warranted leading to appropriate treatment.

Microscopic colitis is a frequent cause of chronic watery diarrhea, especially in older persons. Common associated symptoms include abdominal pain, arthralgias, and weight loss. The incidence of microscopic colitis had been increasing, although more recent studies have shown a stabilization of incidence rates. The diagnosis is based on characteristic histologic findings in a patient with diarrhea. Microscopic colitis can occur at any age, including in children, but it is primarily seen in the elderly. Several treatment options exist to treat the symptoms of microscopic colitis, although only budesonide has been well studied in randomized clinical trials.

The medical management of inflammatory bowel disease (IBD) in the older patient extends beyond luminal disease activity. Factors such as comorbidity, functional status, polypharmacy, and age-related changes in physical reserve and drug metabolism may affect therapeutic decision making. The older patient with IBD is more susceptible to disease-related complications and also to adverse events with therapy, particularly immunosuppression. Appropriate medication selection along with multidisciplinary care, factoring not only disease activity but also these age-related risk factors, may improve therapeutic outcomes and decrease adverse events to therapy.

Clostridium difficile–associated illness is an increasingly prevalent and morbid condition. The elderly population is at a disproportionate risk of developing symptomatic disease and associated complications, including progression to severe or fulminant disease, and development of recurrent infections. This article analyzes the factors that influence *C difficile* disease propensity and severity, with particular attention directed toward features relevant to the rapidly aging population.

Anorectal medical disorders facing the elderly include fecal incontinence, fecal impaction with overflow fecal incontinence, chronic constipation, dyssynergic defecation, hemorrhoids, anal fissure, and pelvic floor disorders. This article discusses the latest advances in age-related changes in morphology and function of anal sphincter, changes in cellular and molecular biology, alterations in neurotransmitters and reflexes, and their impact on functional changes of the anorectum in the elderly. These biophysiologic changes have implications for the pathophysiology of anorectal disorders. A clear understanding and working knowledge of the functional anatomy and pathophysiology will enable appropriate diagnosis and treatment of these disorders.

Constipation is a frequently diagnosed gastrointestinal disorder. Symptoms of constipation are common, with the greatest prevalence in the elderly. Evaluation of constipation begins with a detailed medical history and a focused anorectal examination. Diagnostic testing for constipation is not routinely recommended in the initial evaluation in the absence of alarm signs. Key self-management strategies include increased exercise, a high-fiber diet, and toilet training. High-fiber diets can worsen symptoms in some patients who have chronic constipation. Biofeedback is an effective treatment option for patients who have constipation caused by outlet obstruction defecation. A variety of medications are available to remedy constipation.

Colorectal cancer and precancerous adenomas disproportionately affect the elderly, necessitating the need for screening and surveillance in this group. However, screening and surveillance decisions in the elderly can be challenging. Special considerations such as comorbid medical conditions, functional status, and cognitive ability play a role in one's decisions regarding the utility of screening and surveillance as well as the success and safety of various screening modalities. This article explores the evidence for screening and surveillance in the elderly, and addresses key challenges unique to this population.

There has been limited research examining the risks, benefits, and use of common endoscopic procedures in the elderly. Furthermore, gastroenterology training programs do not routinely incorporate elderly concerns when dealing with common gastrointestinal issues. There exists a broad array of endoscopic procedures with varying inherent risks that must be weighed with each elderly patient in mind. This article discusses the benefits and drawbacks of the most common procedures and indications for endoscopy including upper endoscopy, colonoscopy, endoscopic retrograde cholangiopancreatography, endoscopic ultrasound, percutaneous endoscopic gastrostomy, and deep enteroscopy.

Hepatitis B and hepatitis C are common predisposing factors leading to cirrhosis and liver cancer. Therapies for hepatitis B suppress viral replication and improve morbidity and mortality. Treatment and evaluation of hepatitis B should be similar in all age groups. This article discusses special topics related to hepatitis B and the elderly. Hepatitis C is a treatable disease whose treatment can lead to viral eradication. This article discusses key points regarding hepatitis C diagnosis and treatment in the context of new advances in disease staging and treatment, with special attention on hepatitis C infection in the elderly.

CLINICS IN GERIATRIC MEDICINE

ISSUE OF RELATED INTEREST

Gastroenterology Clinics of North America September 2013 (Vol. 42, No. 3)
Colonoscopy and Polypectomy
Charles J. Kahi, *Editor*
http://www.gastro.theclinics.com/

NOW AVAILABLE FOR YOUR iPhone and iPad

Preface

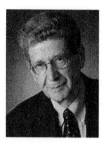

Seymour Katz, MD, FACP, MACG
Editor

The aging patient population presents a multifaceted array of daunting challenges for the clinician. This is particularly true in the management of the older gastroenterologic population faced with medical, procedural, and surgical decisions.

There are several recurrent themes that appear in the following articles in this issue of the *Clinics in Geriatric Medicine*. These include (1) the need to recognize the increasing growth of the elderly population with their unique requirements that will soon comprise 1 of 3 office visits and (2) the impact of a senescent immune system and altered physiology of the elderly. Recognition of changes in body fat, serum proteins, lean body mass, and total body water on plasma concentrations of lipophilic and hydrophilic medications and reduced glomerular filtration rate coupled with impaired medication bioavailabilities and metabolism is a necessary prerequisite to prescribing therapies. (3) The overarching role of multiple comorbidities and polypharmacy with drug-drug interactions further confounds treatment programs. (4) Social factors affecting compliance include altered cognition, mobility, access to support systems, and financial–health insurance restrictions, which add to management concerns. (5) All of the above, when added to the paucity of data and clinical trials involving the elderly, add to the anxiety of creating treatment programs.

Each elderly patient is unique and complex. No "one-size-fits-all" philosophy can be applicable.

Clin Geriatr Med 30 (2014) xiii–xiv
http://dx.doi.org/10.1016/j.cger.2013.10.011
0749-0690/14/$ – see front matter

This volume of detailed "hands-on" information prepared by experienced clinicians is specifically designed to assist the practitioner in the care of the elderly gastroenterologic patient.

Seymour Katz, MD, FACP, MACG
New York University School of Medicine
New York, New York

North Shore University Hospital
Long Island Jewish Hospital System
Manhasset, New York

St. Francis Hospital
Roslyn, New York

1000 Northern Boulevard, Suite 140
Great Neck, NY 11021, USA

E-mail address:
seymourkatz.md@gmail.com

Gastrointestinal Drug Interactions Affecting the Elderly

Mandeep Singh, MD[b], Shawn Chaudhary, MD[b], Sadra Azizi, MD[a], Jesse Green, MD[b],*

KEYWORDS

- Drug interactions • Geriatrics • Common gastrointestinal conditions
- Inflammatory bowel disease • Acid peptic disease • Diarrhea • Constipation
- Endoscopic procedural sedation

KEY POINTS

- This article investigates common interactions between drugs used to treat common geriatric primary care diseases and those used in common gastrointestinal diseases, including acid peptic disease, diarrhea, constipation, endoscopic procedural sedation, and inflammatory bowel disease.
- The predicted exponential growth of elderly patients will create challenging medical management and logistical problems for clinicians.
- This article emphasizes the need for physicians to be vigilant regarding potential drug interactions in a geriatric population burdened with polypharmacy and comorbid conditions.

INTRODUCTION

The United States is undergoing a dramatic shift in demographics. In 2011, people aged 65 years or older accounted for 41.4 million people, or 13.3% of the American population. Since 2000, the elderly population has increased disproportionately to the general population, by 18% versus 9.4%, respectively. Additionally, the number of Americans aged 45 to 64 years who will reach 65 years over the next 2 decades will increase by 33%. By 2030, approximately 72.1 million elderly people will be living in the United States. This exponential growth of elderly patients will create challenging medical management and logistical problems for clinicians.

With the burgeoning elderly population in the United States, drug interactions are an increasing concern because of altered drug metabolism associated with age and polypharmacy. The assessment of drug interactions requires understanding of various age-related factors and issues. This article describes interactions between drugs used in gastrointestinal diseases and those used in geriatric primary care diseases.

[a] Albany Medical Center, Albany, NY, USA; [b] Division of Gastroenterology, Albany Medical Center, Albany, NY, USA
* Corresponding author.
E-mail address: greenj@mail.amc.edu

Clin Geriatr Med 30 (2014) 1–15
http://dx.doi.org/10.1016/j.cger.2013.10.013
0749-0690/14/$ – see front matter © 2014 Elsevier Inc. All rights reserved.

The Lexi-Comp and Epocrates databases were used to analyze possible interactions between various medication classes. PubMed searches were also performed to evaluate recent literature discussing the relationship between common gastrointestinal diseases in the elderly and comorbidities.[1–6]

DRUGS USED IN ACID PEPTIC DISEASES

Elderly patients with severe esophagitis (defined as Los Angeles grade C or D) are at high risk for the development of Barrett esophagus and esophageal adenocarcinoma. Gastroesophageal reflux disease (GERD) in the elderly population often presents with characteristic symptoms, including burning chest discomfort and dysphagia, but may present with uncommon symptoms, including atypical chest pain, severe nausea, and odynophagia. Studies in the elderly population with GERD and esophagitis have shown greater inconsistencies in symptoms as they relate to endoscopic disease severity. In a study of 12,000 patients aged 18 to 75 years with endoscopically documented erosive esophagitis, severe heartburn was seen in 30% of elderly patients aged 70 years or older compared with 47% of younger patients aged 31–40 years. Among these patients, severe esophagitis (defined as Los Angeles grade C or D) was seen in 35% of the elderly patients versus 25% of the younger patients (**Figs. 1 and 2**).[7–9]

Drug classes used in acid peptic disease include antacids, H_2 blockers, proton pump inhibitors, and sucralfate. Each of these agents works by a different mechanism to alter disease process. Lexi-Comp and Epocrates databases were used to analyze interactions between the gastrointestinal drugs calcium carbonate, ranitidine, omeprazole, and Carafate, and those used to treat common elderly diseases, such as hypertension, diabetes, hyperlipidemia, arthritis, and psychiatric illnesses.

Hypertension Medications

Table 1 illustrates interactions between common antihypertensive medications metoprolol, lisinopril, hydrochlorothiazide, furosemide, spironolactone, nifedipine, isosorbide, hydralazine, and losartan, and drugs used in acid peptic disease, such as Tums, ranitidine, omeprazole, and Carafate. As per Epocrates and Lexi-Comp databases, patients taking hydrochlorothiazide and calcium carbonate are at risk of developing hypercalcemia and require close monitoring of serum calcium levels.

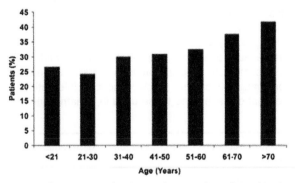

Fig. 1. The prevalence of severe esophagitis and severe heartburn by age decade cohort. (*Data from* Johnson DA, Finnerty MB. Heartburn severity underestimates erosive esophagitis severity in elderly patients with gastroesophageal reflux disease. Gastroenterology 2004;126:660–4.)

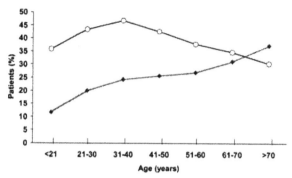

Fig. 2. The prevalence of severe esophagitis by age decade cohort among patients with severe heartburn. (*Data from* Johnson DA, Finnerty MB. Heartburn severity underestimates erosive esophagitis severity in elderly patients with gastroesophageal reflux disease. Gastroenterology 2004;126:660–4.)

Patients taking omeprazole who are also taking furosemide, hydrochlorothiazide, and/or spironolactone have an increased risk of developing hypomagnesemia.

Diabetes Medications

Table 2 illustrates interaction between the diabetes medications metformin, glyburide, rosiglitazone, glargine, intermediate-acting insulin, and pioglitazone, and drugs used in acid peptic disease. Patients using metformin and ranitidine are at risk of having increased metformin levels. As per Epocrates and Lexi-Comp databases, elevated levels of metformin may lead to severe lactic acidosis, especially in patients with underlying renal disease. In patients taking this combination of drugs, baseline renal function should be noted and monitored closely.

Hyperlipidemia Medications

As illustrated in **Table 3**, no significant interaction has been noted between drugs used in acid peptic disease and those used for hyperlipidemia (simvastatin, pravastatin, fenofibrate, niacin, and cholestyramine).

Arthritis/Pain Medications

As per Epocrates and Lexi-Comp databases, the only significant interaction described involving arthritis and pain medications is between enteric-coated naproxen and

Table 1				
Interactions between common medications used for hypertension and acid peptic disease				
	Calcium Carbonate	Ranitidine	Omeprazole	Carafate
Metoprolol	None	None	None	None
Lisinopril	None	None	None	None
Hydrochlorothiazide	Interaction	None	Interaction	None
Furosemide	None	None	Interaction	None
Spironolactone	None	None	Interaction	None
Nifedipine	None	None	None	None
Isosorbide	None	None	None	None
Hydralazine	None	None	None	None
Losartan	None	None	None	None

Table 2
Interactions between common medications used for diabetes and acid peptic disease

	Calcium Carbonate	Ranitidine	Omeprazole	Carafate
Metformin	None	Interaction	None	None
Glyburide	None	None	None	None
Rosiglitazone	None	None	None	None
Glargine	None	None	None	None
Intermediate-acting insulin	None	None	None	None
Pioglitazone	None	None	None	None

omeprazole. This combination can result in the premature dissolution of the enteric coating, causing increase gastrointestinal side effects associated with naproxen (**Table 4**).

Psychotropic Medications

As per Epocrates and Lexi-Comp databases, the only interaction between the outlined psychotropic medications and antisecretory agents listed in **Table 5** is between diazepam and omeprazole. As per Epocrates and Lexi-Comp databases, the concomitant use of a proton pump inhibitor can increase the drug levels of diazepam. Therefore, careful monitoring and dose reduction of the benzodiazepine may be warranted to avoid the risk of oversedation or psychomotor impairment.

CONSTIPATION

Constipation is a common problem in elderly persons, with prevalence ranging from 15% to 20% in the community-dwelling elderly population, and up to 50% in nursing home residents. In the elderly, constipation has a multifactorial cause. Often more than one mechanism is present in a single patient, such as comorbid illnesses or medication side effects. The authors analyzed interactions between drugs used to treat constipation (psyllium, docusate, magnesium hydroxide, lactulose, bisacodyl, lubiprostone, linaclotide) and those used to treat common conditions, such as hypertension, hyperlipidemia, diabetes, arthritis, and psychiatric illnesses.

Hypertension Medications

No significant interaction was observed between drugs commonly used to treat constipation and antihypertensive medications, such as metoprolol, lisinopril, hydrochlorothiazide, furosemide, spironolactone, nifedipine, isosorbide, hydralazine, and losartan (**Table 6**).

Table 3
Interactions between common medications used for hyperlipidemia and acid peptic disease

	Calcium Carbonate	Ranitidine	Omeprazole	Carafate
Simvastatin	None	None	None	None
Pravastatin	None	None	None	None
Fenofibrate	None	None	None	None
Niacin	None	None	None	None
Cholestyramine	None	None	None	None

Table 4
Interactions between common medications used for pain/arthritis and acid peptic disease

	Calcium Carbonate	Ranitidine	Omeprazole	Carafate
Aspirin	None	None	None	None
Naproxen	None	None	Interaction	None
Acetaminophen	None	None	None	None
Tramadol	None	None	None	None
Acetaminophen/codeine	None	None	None	None
Hydrocodone/acetaminophen	None	None	None	None
Morphine	None	None	None	None
Fentanyl	None	None	None	None

Table 5
Interactions between common psychotropic medications and those used in acid peptic disease

	Calcium Carbonate	Ranitidine	Omeprazole	Carafate
Amitriptyline	None	None	None	None
Sertraline	None	None	None	None
Haloperidol	None	None	None	None
Diazepam	None	None	Interaction	None

Table 6
Interactions between common medications used for hypertension and constipation

	Psyllium	Docusate	Lactulose	Magnesium Hydroxide	Bisacodyl	Lubiprostone	Linaclotide
Metoprolol	None	None	None	None	None	None	None
Lisinopril	None	None	None	None	None	None	None
Hydrochlorothiazide	None	None	None	None	None	None	None
Furosemide	None	None	None	None	None	None	None
Spironolactone	None	None	None	None	None	None	None
Nifedipine	None	None	None	None	None	None	None
Isosorbide	None	None	None	None	None	None	None
Hydralazine	None	None	None	None	None	None	None
Losartan	None	None	None	None	None	None	None

Table 7
Interactions between common medications used for diabetes and constipation

	Psyllium	Docusate	Lactulose	Magnesium Hydroxide	Bisacodyl	Lubiprostone	Linaclotide
Metformin	None	None	None	None	None	None	None
Glyburide	None	None	None	None	None	None	None
Rosiglitazone	None	None	None	None	None	None	None
Glargine	None	None	None	None	None	None	None
Intermediate-acting insulin	None	None	None	None	None	None	None
Pioglitazone	None	None	None	None	None	None	None

Diabetes Medications

No significant interactions were seen between drugs commonly used to treat constipation and those used to treat diabetes, such as metformin, glyburide, rosiglitazone, glargine, intermediate-acting insulin, pioglitazone (**Table 7**).

Hyperlipidemia Medications

No significant drug interactions were noted between drugs commonly used to treat constipation and those used to treat hyperlipidemia, such as simvastatin, pravastatin, fenofibrate, niacin, and cholestyramine (**Table 8**).

Arthritis/Pain Medications

Combinations of drugs used to treat arthritis and pain and those used to treat constipation yielded few interactions. As per Epocrates and Lexi-Comp databases, patients using magnesium hydroxide and naproxen are advised to separate administration of these drugs by at least 2 hours, because this combination may predispose to early dissolution of enteric coating, leading to increased gastrointestinal side effects. Caution is also advised with frequent or high-dose antacid use and salicylates, because this combination decreases salicylate levels through enhanced excretion in alkaline urine (**Table 9**).[10–14]

Psychotropic Medications

No significant interactions were noted between psychotropic medications and those used to treat constipation (**Table 10**).[15–17]

DIARRHEA

The prevalence of diarrhea increases with older age, the severity of disability, and the number of drugs taken. Diarrhea can be life-threatening, particularly in patients with multiple comorbidities, immunosenescence, and frailty. Adequate hydration, electrolyte replacement, and infection control should be ensured to avoid complications.[18,19]

Hypertension Medications

Caution is advised when using bismuth/subsalicylate with furosemide, hydrochlorothiazide, metoprolol, lisinopril, and spironolactone. As per Epocrates and Lexi-Comp databases, this combination may decrease antihypertensive, diuretic, and natriuretic efficacy through salicylate-induced inhibition of renal prostaglandins and sodium and water retention. As per Epocrates and Lexi-Comp databases, sublingual nitroglycerine use with anticholinergic medications such as diphenoxylate/atropine may decrease salivary secretions and dissolution of sublingual tablets (**Table 11**).

Table 8
Interactions between common medications used for hyperlipidemia and constipation

	Psyllium	Docusate	Lactulose	Magnesium Hydroxide	Bisacodyl	Lubiprostone	Linaclotide
Simvastatin	None	None	None	None	None	None	None
Pravastatin	None	None	None	None	None	None	None
Fenofibrate	None	None	None	None	None	None	None
Niacin	None	None	None	None	None	None	None
Cholestyramine	None	None	None	None	None	None	None

Table 9
Interactions between common medications used for pain/arthritis and constipation

	Psyllium	Docusate	Lactulose	Magnesium Hydroxide	Bisacodyl	Lubiprostone	Linaclotide
Aspirin	None	None	None	Interaction	None	None	None
Naproxen	None	None	None	Interaction	None	None	None
Acetaminophen	None	None	None	None	None	None	None
Tramadol	None	None	None	None	None	None	None
Acetaminophen/ codeine	None	None	None	None	None	None	None
Hydrocodone/ acetaminophen	None	None	None	None	None	None	None
Morphine	None	None	None	None	None	None	None
Fentanyl	None	None	None	None	None	None	None

Table 10
Interactions between common psychotropic medications and those used in constipation

	Psyllium	Docusate	Lactulose	Magnesium Hydroxide	Bisacodyl	Lubiprostone	Linaclotide
Amitriptyline	None	None	None	None	None	None	None
Sertraline	None	None	None	None	None	None	None
Haloperidol	None	None	None	None	None	None	None
Diazepam	None	None	None	None	None	None	None

Table 11
Interactions between common medications used for hypertension and diarrhea

	Bismuth Subsalicylate	Diphenoxylate/Atropine	Loperamide
Metoprolol	Interaction	None	None
Lisinopril	Interaction	None	None
Hydrochlorothiazide	Interaction	None	None
Furosemide	Interaction	None	None
Spironolactone	Interaction	None	None
Nifedipine	None	None	None
Isosorbide	None	None	None
Hydralazine	None	Interaction	None
Losartan	Interaction	None	None

Table 12
Interactions between common medications used for diabetes and diarrhea

	Bismuth Subsalicylate	Diphenoxylate/Atropine	Loperamide
Metformin	None	None	None
Glyburide	None	None	None
Rosiglitazone	None	None	None
Glargine	None	None	None
Intermediate-acting insulin	None	None	None
Pioglitazone	None	None	None

Diabetes Medications

No significant interaction was observed between drugs used for diabetes (metformin, glyburide, rosiglitazone, glargine, intermediate-acting insulin, pioglitazone) and those used for diarrhea (bismuth, diphenoxylate/atropine, and loperamide) (**Table 12**).

Hyperlipidemia Medications

No significant interaction was observed between drugs used to treat hyperlipidemia (simvastatin, pravastatin, fenofibrate, niacin, cholestyramine) and antidiarrheals (**Table 13**).

Arthritis/Pain Medications

Use of anticholinergics, such as diphenoxylate/atropine and loperamide, with fentanyl, morphine, and acetaminophen/codeine may increase the risk of severe constipation/paralytic ileus. The combination of bismuth and aspirin increases salicylate levels, thereby increasing adverse effects. Bismuth subsalicylate, when used with acetaminophen, acetaminophen/codeine, or hydrocodone/acetaminophen, can result in analgesic-associated nephropathy (**Table 14**).

Psychotropic Medications

As per Epocrates and Lexi-Comp databases, the combination of diphenoxylate/atropine and amitriptyline can potentiate anticholinergic side effects and increase the risk of hyperpyrexia, particularly in patients exposed to high-temperature environments. Anticholinergic side effects are found with diphenoxylate/atropine in conjunction with haloperidol. The use of loperamide in combination with either amitriptyline or haloperidol can increase the risk of severe constipation or paralytic ileus (**Table 15**).

ENDOSCOPIC PROCEDURAL SEDATION

The use of endoscopic procedures has increased in the elderly. Between 2004 and 2008, the incidence of new colorectal cancer diagnoses in the elderly population was 247.6 per 100,000 population compared with 18.2 per 100,000 population in the population younger than 65 years.[20–23] Similarly, elderly patients showed increased rates of esophageal cancer (23.3/100,000 population vs 1.8/100,000 population, respectively) and gastric cancer (40.8/100,000 population vs 3.0/100,000 population, respectively). The elderly also have increased incidences of pancreatic and biliary disease,[24] with gallstones affecting nearly one-third of patients aged 70 years and older.[25]

Table 13
Interactions between common medications used for hyperlipidemia and diarrhea

	Bismuth Subsalicylate	Diphenoxylate/Atropine	Loperamide
Simvastatin	None	None	None
Pravastatin	None	None	None
Fenofibrate	None	None	None
Niacin	None	None	None
Cholestyramine	None	None	None

Table 14
Interactions between common medications used for pain/arthritis and diarrhea

	Bismuth Subsalicylate	Diphenoxylate/Atropine	Loperamide
Aspirin	Interaction	None	None
Naproxen	None	None	None
Acetaminophen	Interaction	None	None
Tramadol	None	None	None
Acetaminophen/codeine	Interaction	None	Interaction
Hydrocodone/acetaminophen	Interaction	None	Interaction
Morphine	None	None	Interaction
Fentanyl	None	Interaction	Interaction

As per Epocrates and Lexi-Comp databases, an increased risk of hypotension, arrhythmias, hypoxia, and aspiration is seen in elderly patients undergoing procedural sedation compared with the younger population. In 2006, the American Society of Gastrointestinal Endoscopy issued guidelines regarding the use of sedation in elderly patients undergoing endoscopic procedures.[26] Because of physiologic changes associated with aging, the guidelines recommend using fewer sedative agents at lower doses than in younger patients, and administering the medications with slower infusion rates.

Hypertension Medications

Drugs such as metoprolol, lisinopril, hydrochlorothiazide, furosemide, spironolactone, isosorbide, hydralazine, and losartan have no significant interactions with drugs used for procedural sedation, such as midazolam, fentanyl, and propofol. However, as per Epocrates and Lexi-Comp databases, the combination of nifedipine and fentanyl may increase the risk of hypotension (**Table 16**).

Diabetes Medications

As per Epocrates and Lexi-Comp databases, the combination of pioglitazone and midazolam can decrease levels of midazolam, resulting in decreased efficacy. No significant interaction was observed with other diabetes medications, including metformin, glyburide, rosiglitazone, glargine, and intermediate-acting insulin (**Table 17**).

Hyperlipidemia Medications

No significant interaction occurs with drugs used to treat hyperlipidemia (simvastatin, pravastatin, fenofibrate, niacin, cholestyramine) and those used for procedural sedation (**Table 18**).

Table 15
Interactions between common psychotropic medications and those used in diarrhea

	Bismuth Subsalicylate	Diphenoxylate/Atropine	Loperamide
Amitriptyline	None	Interaction	Interaction
Sertraline	None	None	None
Haloperidol	None	Interaction	Interaction
Diazepam	None	None	None

Table 16
Interactions between common medications used for hypertension and those used in procedural sedation

	Midazolam	Fentanyl	Propofol
Metoprolol	None	None	None
Lisinopril	None	None	None
Hydrochlorothiazide	None	None	None
Furosemide	None	None	None
Spironolactone	None	None	None
Nifedipine	None	Interaction	None
Isosorbide	None	None	None
Hydralazine	None	None	None
Losartan	None	None	None

Table 17
Interactions between common medications used for diabetes and those used in procedural sedation

	Midazolam	Fentanyl	Propofol
Simvastatin	None	None	None
Pravastatin	None	None	None
Fenofibrate	None	None	None
Niacin	None	None	None
Cholestyramine	None	None	None

Table 18
Interactions between common medications used for hyperlipidemia and those used in procedural sedation

	Midazolam	Fentanyl	Propofol
Aspirin	None	None	None
Naproxen	None	None	None
Acetaminophen	None	None	None
Tramadol	Interaction	Interaction	Interaction
Acetaminophen/codeine	Interaction	Interaction	Interaction
Hydrocodone/acetaminophen	Interaction	Interaction	Interaction
Morphine	Interaction	Interaction	Interaction
Fentanyl	Interaction	N/A	Interaction

Abbreviation: N/A, not applicable.

Arthritis/Pain Medications

As per Epocrates and Lexi-Comp databases, propofol combined with acetamino-phen/codeine, hydrocodone/acetaminophen, and tramadol may result in profound central nervous system (CNS) and respiratory depression. An increased risk of sei-zures is possible with the combination of tramadol and fentanyl (**Table 19**).

Psychotropic Medications

As per Epocrates and Lexi-Comp databases, midazolam in combination with amitrip-tyline, haloperidol, or diazepam can increase the risk of CNS depression. When used with fentanyl, diazepam can have similar effects, including oversedation and psycho-motor impairment, and can result in vasodilation and subsequent hypotension. Addi-tive effects of sertraline with diazepam can increase the risk of serotonin syndrome or neuroleptic malignant syndrome. Fentanyl with amitriptyline places patients at risk for serotonin syndrome, CNS depression, psychomotor impairment, and severe consti-pation. Propofol in conjunction with amitriptyline, haloperidol, or diazepam can in-crease the risk for oversedation, respiratory depression, and hypotension (**Table 20**).

INFLAMMATORY BOWEL DISEASE

Inflammatory bowel disease is known to have a bimodal distribution with respect to age of onset, with 15% of cases presenting at or older than 65 years. The Epocrates database was used to analyze interactions between various drugs used by elderly patients.[27,28]

Hypertension Medications

As per Epocrates and Lexi-Comp databases, few interactions have been reported be-tween antihypertensive medications and drugs used to treat inflammatory bowel dis-ease. Prednisone taken with either furosemide or hydrochlorothiazide increases hypokalemia through additive effects of both medications, and thus potassium levels must be monitored. An antagonist effect occurs between the 2 medications, resulting in decreased efficacy of the diuretic. Dose adjustment of the diuretic or switching to a different class of antihypertensives is necessary. Azathioprine and lisinopril can in-crease the risk for severe leucopenia through an unclear mechanism (**Table 21**).

Diabetic Medications

As per Epocrates and Lexi-Comp databases, the hyperglycemia caused by cortico-steroids will decrease the efficacy of the diabetic medication in question, and patients often require a dose escalation or additional medications to provide adequate

Table 19 Interactions between common medications used for pain/arthritis and those used in procedural sedation			
	Midazolam	**Fentanyl**	**Propofol**
Metformin	None	None	None
Glyburide	None	None	None
Rosiglitazone	None	None	None
Glargine	None	None	None
Intermediate-acting insulin	None	None	None
Pioglitazone	Interaction	None	None

Table 20
Interactions between common psychotropic medications and those used in procedural sedation

	Midazolam	Fentanyl	Propofol
Amitriptyline	Interaction	Interaction	Interaction
Sertraline	None	Interaction	None
Haloperidol	Interaction	None	Interaction
Diazepam	Interaction	Interaction	None

glycemic control. Lactic acidosis may occur with increased levels of metformin when combined with either mesalamine or methotrexate (**Table 22**).

Hyperlipidemia Medications

As per Epocrates and Lexi-Comp databases, prednisone in combination with cholestyramine results in decreased corticosteroid levels and efficacy from decreased absorption. Cholestyramine, a bile-acid binding resin, affects the absorption of prednisone, and therefore corticosteroids should be given either 1 or more hours before or 4 to 6 hours after cholestyramine administration. Infliximab given with simvastatin results in decreased drugs levels and efficacy of simvastatin because of the biologics downregulation of the hepatic CYP450 enzyme (**Table 23**).

Arthritis/Pain Medications

As per Epocrates and Lexi-Comp databases, the combination of prednisone with either aspirin or naproxen increases the risk of gastrointestinal bleeding. Prednisone may reduce aspirin levels and thus its efficacy. The additive effects of prednisone and naproxen can lead to sodium and water retention and resulting edema. Aspirin in high doses can increase methotrexate drug levels with related toxicities. This effect is of particular concern in elderly patients, especially those with renal insufficiency. Blood counts of patients on this combination of drugs should be carefully checked. Methotrexate and naproxen use warrants monitoring for methotrexate toxicity and requires serial blood counts. Aspirin given with mesalamine can increase the risk of salicylate toxicity. Infliximab use with either fentanyl or tramadol can result in decreased drug levels and efficacy of either of these pain medications because of infliximab's effects on the hepatic CYP450 enzyme pathway (**Table 24**).

Table 21
Interactions between common medications used for hypertension and inflammatory bowel disease

	Prednisone	Mesalamine	Mercaptopurine	Azathioprine	Infliximab	Methotrexate
Metoprolol	None	None	None	None	None	None
Lisinopril	None	None	None	Interaction	None	None
Hydrochlorothiazide	Interaction	None	None	None	None	None
Lasix	Interaction	None	None	None	None	None
Spironolactone	None	None	None	None	None	None
Nifedipine	None	None	None	None	None	None
Isosorbide	None	None	None	None	None	None
Hydralazine	None	None	None	None	None	None
Losartan	None	None	None	None	None	None

Table 22

Interactions between common medications used for diabetes and inflammatory bowel disease

	Prednisone	Mesalamine	Mercaptopurine	Azathioprine	Infliximab	Methotrexate
Metformin	Interaction	Interaction	None	None	None	Interaction
Glyburide	Interaction	None	None	None	None	None
Rosiglitazone	None	None	None	None	None	None
Glargine	Interaction	None	None	None	None	None
Intermediate-acting insulin	Interaction	None	None	None	None	None
Pioglitazone	Interaction	None	None	None	None	None

Table 23

Interactions between common medications used for hyperlipidemia and inflammatory bowel disease

	Prednisone	Mesalamine	Mercaptopurine	Azathioprine	Infliximab	Methotrexate
Simvastatin	None	None	None	None	Interaction	None
Pravastatin	None	None	None	None	None	None
Fenofibrate	None	None	None	None	None	None
Niacin	None	None	None	None	None	None
Cholestyramine	Interaction	None	None	None	None	None

Table 24

Interactions between common medications used for pain/arthritis and inflammatory bowel disease

	Prednisone	Mesalamine	Mercaptopurine	Azathioprine	Infliximab	Methotrexate
Aspirin	Interaction	Interaction	None	None	None	Interaction
Naproxen	Interaction	None	None	None	None	Interaction
Tylenol	None	None	None	None	None	None
Tramadol	None	None	None	None	Interaction	None
Percocet	None	None	None	None	None	None
Vicodin	None	None	None	None	None	None
Morphine	None	None	None	None	None	None
Fentanyl	None	None	None	None	Interaction	None

Table 25

Interactions between common psychotropic medications and those used in inflammatory bowel disease

	Prednisone	Mesalamine	Mercaptopurine	Azathioprine	Infliximab	Methotrexate
Amitriptyline	None	None	None	None	Interaction	None
Sertraline	None	None	None	None	None	None
Haloperidol	Interaction	None	None	None	Interaction	None
Diazepam	None	None	None	None	None	None

Psychotropic Medications

As per Epocrates and Lexi-Comp databases, hypokalemia can result when predni-sone is taken with haloperidol, along with QT prolongation and cardiac arrhythmias. Infliximab can decrease levels of amitriptyline and haloperidol, potentially reducing the inefficacy **(Table 25)**.

SUMMARY

As the geriatric population increases in the United States, greater attention must be directed to common drug interactions. This article emphasizes the need for physicians to be vigilant regarding potential drug interactions in a geriatric population burdened with polypharmacy and comorbid conditions.

REFERENCES

1. U.S. Census Bureau. Statistical Abstract of the United States. 2012.
2. American Geriatrics Society 2012 Beers Criteria Update Expert Panel. American Geriatrics Society updated Beers criteria for potentially inappropriate medication use in older adults. J Am Geriatr Soc 2012;10:1532–41.
3. Steinman MA, Handler SM, Gurwitz JH, et al. Beyond the prescription: medication monitoring and adverse drug events in older adults. J Am Geriatr Soc 2011;59: 1513–20.
4. Chutka DS, Evans JM, Fleming KC, et al. Drug prescribing for elderly patients. Mayo Clin Proc 1995;70:685–93.
5. Long SH. Prescription drugs and the elderly: issues and options. Health Aff 1994; 13(2):157–74.
6. Hall KE, Proctor DD, Fisher L, et al. American Gastroenterological Association future trends committee reports: effects of aging of the population on gastroen-terology practice, education and research. Gastroenterology 2005;129: 1305–38.
7. Zhu H, Pace F, Sangaletti O, et al. Features of symptomatic gastroesophageal reflux in elderly patients. Scand J Gastroenterol 1993;28:235–8.
8. Collen MJ, Abdulian JD, Chen YK. Gastroesophageal reflux disease in the elderly: more severe disease that requires aggressive therapy. Am J Gastroen-terol 1995;90:1053–7.
9. Johnson DA, Finnerty MB. Heartburn severity underestimates erosive esophagitis severity in elderly patients with gastroesophageal reflux disease. Gastroenter-ology 2004;126:660–4.
10. American Gastroenterological Association. American Gastroenterological Associ-ation medical position statement: guidelines on constipation. Gastroenterology 2000;119:1761–78.
11. Feinberg M. The problems of anticholinergic adverse effects in older patients. Drugs Aging 1993;3(4):335–48.
12. Harari D, Gurwitz JH, Minaker KL. Constipation in the elderly. J Am Geriatr Soc 1993;41(10):1130–40.
13. Tune L, Carr S, Hoag E, et al. Anticholinergic effects of drugs commonly pre-scribed for the elderly: potential means for assessing risk of delirium. Am J Psy-chiatry 1992;149(10):1393–4.
14. Locke GR 3rd, Pemberton JH, Phillips SF. AGA technical review on constipation. American Gastroenterological Association. Gastroenterology 2000;119(6): 1766–78.

15. Locke GR 3rd, Pemberton JH, Phillips SF. American Gastroenterological Association medical position statement: guide lines on constipation. Gastroenterology 2000;119(6):1761–6.

16. Talley NJ, O'Keefe EA, Zinsmeister AR, et al. Prevalence of gastrointestinal symptoms in the elderly: a population-based study. Gastroenterology 1992;102: 895–901.

17. O'Keefe EA, Talley NJ, Zinsmeister AR, et al. Bowel disorders impair functional status and quality of life in the elderly: a population-based study. J Gerontol A Biol Sci Med Sci 1995;50:M184–9.

18. Lew JF, Glass RI, Gangarosa RE, et al. Diarrheal deaths in the United States, 1979 through 1987. A special problem for the elderly. JAMA 1991;265:3280–4.

19. Faruque AS, Malek MA, Khan AI, et al. Diarrhoea in elderly people: aetiology and clinical characteristics. Scand J Infect Dis 2004;36:204–8.

20. Mönkemüller K, Fry LC, Malfertheiner P, et al. Gastrointestinal endoscopy in the elderly: current issues. Best Pract Res Clin Gastroenterol 2009;23:821–7.

21. Qureshi WA, Zuckerman MJ, Adler DG, et al, Standards of Practice Committee, American Society for Gastrointestinal Endoscopy. ASGE guideline: modifications in endoscopic practice for the elderly. Gastrointest Endosc 2006;63:566–9.

22. Beekman AT, Copeland JR, Prince MJ. Review of community prevalence of depression in later life. Br J Psychiatry 1999;174:307.

23. Shrestha LB. CRS report for congress. Life expectancy in the United States. Available at: http://aging.senate.gov/crs/aging1.pdf. Accessed February 13, 2012.

24. Hutchison LC, O'Brien CE. Changes in pharmacokinetics and pharmacodynamics in the elderly patient. J Pharm Pract 2007;20:4–12.

25. Mangoni AA, Jackson SH. Age-related changes in pharmacokinetics and pharmacodynamics: basic principles and practical applications. Br J Clin Pharmacol 2004;57:6–14.

26. Manabe N, Yoshihara M, Sasaki A, et al. Clinical characteristics and natural history of patients with low-grade reflux esophagitis. J Gastroenterol Hepatol 2002; 17:949–54.

27. Robertson DJ, Grimm IS. Inflammatory bowel disease in the elderly. Gastroenterol Clin North Am 2001;30:409–26.

28. Manten E, Green J, Bartholomew C. Primary care consideration in the management of inflammatory bowel disease patients. Pract Gastroenterol 2012;36:48–54.

Vaccinations in Older Adults with Gastrointestinal Diseases

Henry A. Horton, MD, Hayoon Kim, MD, Gil Y. Melmed, MD, MS*

KEYWORDS

- Vaccination • Prophylaxis • Gastrointestinal diseases • Inflammatory bowel disease
- Cirrhosis • Hepatitis • Zoster • Influenza

KEY POINTS

- Older adults (age ≥65 years) have decreased response rates to most vaccines.
- Patients with chronic gastrointestinal diseases, including chronic liver disease and inflammatory bowel disease, are at increased risk of infections, and generally respond less robustly to vaccines.
- Vaccination status should be assessed and appropriate vaccines administered in the older adult population with chronic gastrointestinal diseases, who are more susceptible to vaccine-preventable illnesses than their younger counterparts.
- Special vaccination considerations for older adults with chronic gastrointestinal diseases include the potential use of double-dose influenza vaccination, avoidance of the live influenza vaccine, and special considerations for the herpes zoster vaccine at the age of 60 and older.

INTRODUCTION

According to the 2012 census, 13.7% of the United States population is older than 65 years. It is projected that by 2050, nearly 35% of the population in the will be over that age.[1] Improvements in health care treatment and prevention, including vaccinations, have led to an increase in the average life expectancy worldwide, especially in industrialized nations.[1] Vaccines are a cost-effective and efficient way of preventing morbidity and mortality caused by infectious disease.[2] Because the efficacy of a vaccine depends on the quality of the patient's immune system, the elderly and patients who are immunocompromised are frequently not as protected by vaccinations as the general population.[3] Multiple recent studies have shown that elderly patients (generally defined as those older than 60 years), particularly those older than

Division of Gastroenterology, Department of Medicine, Cedars-Sinai Medical Center, Los Angeles, CA 90048, USA
* Corresponding author. 8730 Alden Drive, 203 West, Thalians Building, IBD Center, Los Angeles, CA 90048.
E-mail address: melmedg@cshs.org

Clin Geriatr Med 30 (2014) 17–28
http://dx.doi.org/10.1016/j.cger.2013.10.002
0749-0690/14/$ – see front matter © 2014 Elsevier Inc. All rights reserved.

75, have decreased immune responses to vaccines in comparison with individuals who are 60 to 74 years of age and even less than those below the age of 60.[3,4] Given the aging population, more patients with chronic gastrointestinal illnesses, including chronic liver disease (viral hepatitis, cirrhosis, autoimmune hepatitis) and inflammatory bowel disease (Crohn disease and ulcerative colitis), will face the challenge of diseases that may compromise their ability to fight various infections, as well a natural age-related decline in their immune system that may decrease the effectiveness of vaccinations.

ELDERLY RESPONSE TO VACCINATION

The age-related decline in the immune response is called immunosenescence, which results from several changes in the immune system that occur as people get older, including changes in the function of antigen-presenting cells, loss of native T cells, and reduced B-cell affinity, production, and half-lives (**Fig. 1** and **Table 1**).[5–14] Furthermore, they have an increased likelihood of vaccine-preventable infections, and are more apt to experience greater severity of influenza, meningitis, pneumococcal pneumonia, tetanus, and herpes zoster.[3,7,9] These infections can also exacerbate underlying comorbidities in the elderly, leading to worse outcomes.[15]

CLINICAL VIGNETTES
Case 1

A 68-year-old man with mildly elevated liver enzymes undergoes evaluation and is found to have a new diagnosis of hepatitis C cirrhosis. What vaccinations should be considered?

Case 2

A 71-year-old practicing physician with ulcerative colitis on azathioprine (2.5 mg/kg daily) inquires about what vaccines she should receive. What do you recommend?

VACCINATION PRINCIPLES FOR PERSONS OF AGE 60 AND OLDER

In general, the adult schedule for vaccinations should be followed for all patients with chronic gastrointestinal conditions, similar to those without chronic illnesses, with a few specific differences as noted in **Table 2**. The vaccines for which older age marks a change from recommendations in younger people include measles-mumps-rubella (MMR) vaccine, pneumococcal vaccination, and zoster vaccination. Influenza vaccination is discussed here as well, given the very significant impact of this seasonal infection on those aged 65 years and older.

MMR Vaccination

The MMR vaccine is only indicated for individuals born in 1957 or later without childhood vaccination, as all those born before 1957 are generally considered immune. An exception to the rule is for health care providers born before 1957, who do require revaccination with MMR if they do not have serologic evidence of immunity to measles, mumps, or rubella.

Pneumococcal Vaccination

The 23-valent pneumococcal polysaccharide vaccine (PSV23; Pneumovax) is recommended for all adults age 65 years or older. Furthermore, patients who have previously

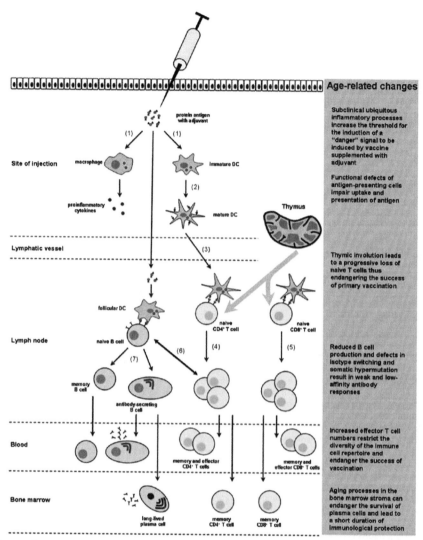

Fig. 1. The immune response and its age-related alterations following vaccination. Protein antigens administered together with adjuvants induce the activations of innate immune responses at the site of injection. The antigen is taken up by antigen-presenting cells, such as macrophages and dendritic cells (DCs). The local innate immune response facilitates maturation of DCs, which present stable major histocompatibility complex/peptide complexes. Mature DCs migrate into lymph nodes, where they induce activation and clonal expansion of naïve CD4+ and CD8+ T cells. The activation and differentiation of naïve B cells is induced by antigen and CD4+ T-cell help. Naïve B cells differentiate into memory B cells and antibody-secreting B cells. Long-term immunity is assured by memory B and T cells in the blood and lymph nodes, as well as by long-lived plasma cells and memory T cells in the bone marrow. (*From* Weinberger B, Herndler-Brandstetter D, Schwanninger A, et al. Biology of immune responses to vaccines in elderly persons. Clin Infect Dis 2008;46(7):1078–84; with permission.)

Table 1
Vaccines and their efficacy in elderly persons

Disease	Vaccine Type	Vaccine Efficacy in Elderly Persons (%)
Influenza		
A/H1N1	Inactivated virus, subunit, adjuvanted subunit, and virosome	55 (32)[a]
A/H3N2	Inactivated virus, subunit, adjuvanted subunit, and virosome	58 (46)[a]
B	Inactivated virus, subunit, adjuvanted subunit, and virosome	41 (29)[a]
Hepatitis		
A	Inactivated virus	63[b]
A	Virosome	65 (97)[c]
B	Subunit	33[b]
Herpes zoster	Live attenuated virus	64 (18)[d]
Pertussis	Toxoid and acellular components	>81[e]
Pneumonia	Nonconjugated polysaccharide	50–70[f]
Poliomyelitis	Inactivated virus	99[g]
Tetanus and diphtheria	Toxoid	99 and 84[h]
Tickborne encephalitis	Inactivated virus	70[i]
Yellow fever	Live attenuated virus	100

[a] Seroprotection of persons aged 65–74 years ($\geq$75 years).
[b] Seroprotection (antihepatitis A virus concentration $\geq$20 IU/L; antihepatitis B surface antigen concentration of $\geq$10 IU/L) of persons aged $\geq$60 years after 2 booster vaccinations.
[c] Seroprotection ($\geq$20 IU/L) of persons aged $\geq$50 years after primary vaccination (after booster vaccination).
[d] Vaccine efficacy in persons aged 60–69 years ($\geq$80 years old).
[e] Elderly persons (median age, 66 years) with protective antibody levels against pertussis after vaccination with low-dose diphtheria, tetanus, pertussis, and inactivated poliovirus vaccine.
[f] Vaccine efficacy in the general elderly population regarding invasive pneumococcal disease.
[g] Vaccine efficacy in elderly persons (median age, 66 years) after booster vaccination with low-dose diphtheria, tetanus, pertussis, and inactivated poliovirus vaccine.
[h] Elderly persons (median age, 66 years) with protective antibody levels against tetanus and diphtheria after booster vaccination with low-dose diphtheria, tetanus, pertussis, and inactivated poliovirus vaccine.
[i] Elderly persons (>60 years) with protective antibody levels ($\geq$100 Vienna units/mL) against tickborne encephalitis after booster vaccination 3–4 years after the last vaccination.

Data from Refs.[7–14]; and *Reprinted from* Weinberger B, Herndler-Brandstetter D, Schwanninger A, et al. Biology of immune responses to vaccines in elderly persons. Clin Infect Dis 2008;46:1079; with permission.

received 1 or 2 doses of PSV23 for any reason should receive another dose at the age of 65 or older, provided that 5 years have elapsed since the last dose.

It is increasingly apparent that the effectiveness of pneumococcal vaccination among the elderly is in doubt. Epidemiologic studies have not clearly demonstrated that pneumococcal vaccination reduces pneumonia specifically in the elderly population. Historically, PSV23 has been recommended for older adults; however, new developments in vaccine immunogenicity, such as the 13-valent pneumococcal conjugate vaccine (PCV13) (now approved for adults in the United States) may provide improved efficacy, perhaps in combination with the broader coverage offered by PSV23.[16] At present, however, age alone does not warrant consideration for the PCV13 vaccine,

Table 2
Vaccination recommendations for adults age 65 years or older

	General Recommendations	Recommendations for Those with Chronic Liver Disease	Recommendations for Those with IBD/on Immunosuppressive Therapy
Influenza	Annual standard-dose or high-dose inactivated influenza vaccine	Annual standard-dose or high-dose inactivated influenza vaccine	Annual standard-dose or high-dose inactivated influenza vaccine[a]
Tetanus, diphtheria, pertussis	Get a Tdap once, then a Td booster every 10 y	Get a Tdap once, then a Td booster every 10 y	Get a Tdap once, then a Td booster every 10 y[a]
Varicella	Two doses, if not immune	Two doses, if not immune	Do not give if immunosuppressed
Zoster	One dose (age 60)	One dose (age 60)	Consider on a case-by-case basis (see text)
Measles, mumps, rubella (MMR)	N/A[b]	N/A[b]	N/A[b], but do not give if immunosuppressed
Pneumococcal polysaccharide (PSV23)	One dose at age 65[c]	One dose at age 65[c]	One dose at age 65[a,c]
Hepatitis A	If specific risk factors[d]	Two doses	If specific risk factors[a,d]
Hepatitis B	If specific risk factors[e]	Two doses	If specific risk factors[a,e,f]
Meningococcal	If specific risk factors[g]	If specific risk factors[g]	If specific risk factors[g]

Abbreviation: N/A, not applicable.

[a] People with IBD (at all ages) have diminished immune responses to these vaccines if on combination therapy with anti-TNF and immunomodulator; if possible try to administer before immunosuppression.

[b] MMR is not generally given to older adults, except in the case of health care providers without documented evidence of immunity to measles, mumps, or rubella.

[c] Persons who received 1 or 2 doses of PSV23 before age 65 for any indication should receive another dose of the vaccine at age 65 years or later if at least 5 years have elapsed since the previous dose.

[d] Risk factors warranting hepatitis A vaccination include: men who have sex with men, people who anticipate close personal contact with someone from an endemic area, travelers to endemic areas.

[e] Risk factors warranting hepatitis B vaccination include: sexually active people not in mutually monogamous relationships, people seeking evaluation for sexually transmitted disease, men who have sex with men, health care personnel, persons with diabetes with need for blood glucose monitoring in a long-term care facility, persons with end-stage renal disease or receiving hemodialysis, close contacts of individuals with hepatitis B surface antigen positive, adults in facilities providing human immunodeficiency virus testing, treatment for sexually transmitted disease, services to injection drug users, daycare facilities for people with developmental disabilities; anyone who wants one.

[f] Double doses of hepatitis B vaccine at the usual 3-dose interval is associated with improved vaccine response rates.

[g] Risk factors warranting meningococcal vaccination include microbiologists exposed to *Neisseria meningitides*, military recruits, and persons living in/traveling to endemic areas.

Adapted from www.cdc.gov/vaccines/schedules/hcp/imz/adult.html. Accessed September 1, 2013.

which is more immunogenic in young children and is recommended for adults with compromised immunity.

Zoster Vaccination

Vaccination against herpes zoster is approved for adults 50 and older. Of note, this is a live-virus vaccine with implications for those with compromised immunity or on immunosuppressive therapies, for whom live vaccines are generally contraindicated. Zoster vaccination (see later discussion) is one of the most important vaccines to consider in any older individual, but particularly in those individuals with chronic illnesses who may be at increased risk for herpes zoster, complications thereof (eye involvement, disseminated disease, hospitalization), and post-herpetic neuralgia.

Influenza Vaccination

More than 90% of influenza-related deaths occur among people older than 60 years.[17] This risk is compounded when older adults have chronic gastrointestinal illnesses. For example, patients with cirrhosis (at any age) have increased morbidity associated with influenza infection, including increased rates of hepatic failure and hospitalization.[18] The trivalent inactivated influenza vaccine should be given yearly as is recommended for all adults, although the live, attenuated influenza vaccine is not recommended to anyone older than 49 years.

Despite studies showing decreased antibody response after vaccination in the elderly,[8,19] recommendations for influenza vaccination among elderly adults do not currently differ from those for younger adults, other than avoidance of the live intranasal vaccine. However, strategies to improve vaccine response rates are being investigated. In 2010 the Fluzone high dose (containing 4 times the amount of influenza strains as the regular dose) was licensed for adults aged 65 years and older. Evidence associating higher vaccine responses using this high-dose vaccine with lower rates of influenza infections and complications are still forthcoming. Current recommendations give the option of the normal-dose or the high-dose inactivated vaccine for adults of age 65 and older.

HEPATITIS C, CHRONIC LIVER DISEASE, AND INFECTIONS IN THE ELDERLY
Hepatitis C Virus

Hepatitis C virus (HCV) is a common cause of morbidity and mortality in the United States, and a common cause of chronic liver disease, eventually leading to cirrhosis.[20,21] The Centers for Disease Control and Prevention estimate that although persons born between 1945 and 1965 comprise an estimated 27% of the United States population, they account for 75% of all HCV infections and 73% of all HCV-associated mortality. Therefore, recent US Preventive Services Task Force guidelines recommend screening for hepatitis C in all adults born from 1945 to 1965, the "baby boomer" generation. Although most of these individuals are currently younger than 65 years, they will represent an increasingly larger segment of the population at risk for preventable infections over the coming years. This population is also at greater risk than their young counterparts for hepatocellular carcinoma and other HCV-related liver disease.[22]

Acute hepatitis A and B are rarely fatal in healthy adults but can cause acute liver failure and death in patients with chronic hepatitis C, particularly the elderly.[23,24] Thus it is recommended that all adults with hepatitis C receive vaccination against hepatitis A and B if they are not already vaccinated.[25] However, vaccine responses to hepatitis A and B are often inadequate in the elderly, theoretically resulting in suboptimal protection. Thus in elderly patients with HCV, one should consider monitoring antibodies to hepatitis A and B vaccines, because booster doses (extra doses) or double doses of the vaccines have been shown to be effective in boosting immunity.[22–24]

Autoimmune Hepatitis

Although generally thought of as a disease of younger women, autoimmune hepatitis can affect men and women of any age. In fact, elderly individuals make up roughly 25% of all cases of autoimmune hepatitis.[26,27] Autoimmune hepatitis is characterized by circulating autoantibodies and a high serum γ-globulin concentration.[26] Like any type of chronic liver disease, autoimmune hepatitis can lead to fibrosis and, eventually, cirrhosis and liver failure. Chronic immunosuppression is the mainstay of therapy, and may include corticosteroids, azathioprine, and 6-mercaptopurine.[26] Similar to other autoimmune diseases that require the use of immunosuppressive therapies, it is reasonable to extrapolate that patients with autoimmune hepatitis on immunosuppression will also not have an inadequate response to certain vaccines.[27,28] Thus vaccination, particularly against hepatitis A and B, is recommended in patients with autoimmune hepatitis, ideally before initiating immunosuppressive therapy, as patients have worse outcomes if they develop either infection. This aspect is particularly true in the elderly, who tend to be diagnosed with autoimmune hepatitis at a later stage of disease than their younger counterparts and often have a more severe disease course.[29] Furthermore, the increased risk of infections associated with the use of corticosteroids and thiopurines warrants adherence to age-appropriate guidelines for vaccination against influenza, pneumococcal infection, and herpes zoster among patients with autoimmune hepatitis who are older than 60 years.

Chronic Liver Disease and Cirrhosis

Chronic liver disease from any cause, and resultant cirrhosis, are increasingly common in the elderly. In developed countries, common causes of chronic liver disease and cirrhosis in the elderly include chronic viral hepatitis (B and C), alcoholic liver disease, and autoimmune hepatitis.[20,21]

Cirrhosis represents a late stage of chronic liver disease characterized by progressive and often irreversible hepatic fibrosis. Patients with cirrhosis are at risk of developing infections resulting from altered immune defenses.[30,31] The liver plays a key role in innate immunity, primarily because of its encounter of ingested pathogens through the enterohepatic circulation.[31] Cirrhotic patients have hepatic dysfunction attributable to senescence of the reticuloendothelial system (Kupffer cells, macrophages, and monocytes) as well as dysfunctional neutrophils, eosinophils, and basophils.[31] Increased gut permeability of bacteria and associated toxins in patients with cirrhosis can lead to spontaneous infections.[32] Cirrhosis also results in extensive shunting of venous circulation away from the liver, thus impairing the normal clearing capacity after infection. Patients with cirrhosis are thus at increased risk for infections, many of which are preventable with vaccinations including bacterial pneumococcal infections causing pneumonia, bacteremia and meningitis, and viral infections such as influenza and herpes zoster.

Patients older than 65 with cirrhosis have even worse outcomes than their younger counterparts, owing to an overall higher risk of complications, many of which relate to a higher risk of infections in the general elderly population, decreased responsiveness to vaccines, and systemic comorbidities that compound risks for and from infections.[32,33]

Summary of Vaccine Recommendations for Elderly Patients with Advanced Liver Disease and Cirrhosis

Vaccination recommendations for elderly patients with chronic liver disease or cirrhosis are similar to those for healthy individuals, with a few exceptions. These recommendations include vaccination against hepatitis A and B, which should be given as soon as possible after the diagnosis of chronic liver disease, as well as pneumococcal vaccination with the 23-valent vaccine (even if previously received, provided that the last dose was at least 5 years prior). Assessment of postvaccination titers may help identify patients who may benefit from additional doses of vaccine. Influenza vaccination should be given annually, and herpes zoster vaccination should be given to all adults older than 60 with chronic liver disease, as per routine guidelines.

INFLAMMATORY BOWEL DISEASE

Inflammatory bowel disease (IBD) is characterized by dysregulation of the immune system that is triggered inappropriately by commensal gut bacteria, resulting in an overly active intestinal immune response. IBD includes both ulcerative colitis and Crohn disease. The treatment of IBD frequently involves the use of immunosuppressive medications, namely glucocorticoids, immune modulators (including azathioprine, 6-mercaptopurine, and methotrexate), and tumor necrosis factor (TNF)-α inhibitors such as infliximab (Remicade), adalimumab (Humira), golimumab (Simponi), and certolizumab (Cimzia). As a result of this immunosuppression, patients with IBD are at higher risk for vaccine-preventable infections including varicella, zoster, pneumococcal pneumonia, and influenza.[34]

Although IBD typically affects younger people, it can be diagnosed at any age, with an increasing prevalence of IBD among adults aged 65 years and older. There is increasing awareness of special concerns among this growing population, particularly related to infectious risks that increase with age and are compounded by both the disease and commonly used immunosuppressive treatments. Furthermore, the "polypharmacy" use of multiple medications in the elderly raises the potential for drug-drug interactions that could render patients even more susceptible to infections through hepatotoxicity, nephrotoxicity, and bone marrow suppression.

Vaccine recommendations for persons with IBD who are older than 65 do not differ significantly from guidelines for those younger than 65 years (see the section on vaccination principles). However, a discussion of herpes zoster infection and vaccination is warranted, given the high risk and significant morbidity associated with this infection in both the elderly and the general IBD population.

Vaccine Responses in IBD

Several studies have evaluated the impact of IBD therapies on various vaccine response rates, although no published studies have specifically looked at response rates among older individuals. An emerging theme from several of these studies is that patients with IBD who are on combination therapy (azathioprine or 6-mercaptopurine together with a TNF inhibitor) have significantly decreased immunologic responses to several vaccines in comparison with those not on combination therapy,[28,34] whereas those on monotherapy with a thiopurine or anti-TNF agent generally respond normally to commonly administered vaccines. In the elderly patient with an already diminished likelihood of vaccine response and protection, it is therefore reasonable to assess postvaccination titers and to administer extra booster doses when they are low.[34,35]

Herpes Zoster Vaccine

Herpes zoster infection, also known as shingles, causes a painful, blistering rash usually isolated to single or adjacent dermatomes. Complications include post-herpetic neuralgia in roughly 15% of patients, which can last months to years after initial infection without effective treatments. Other complications include bacterial superinfections and viral meningitis. People aged 60 years and older are 3 to 7 times more likely to develop herpes zoster infection than those who are younger. Immunocompromised patients, including those with IBD, are twice as likely to develop herpes zoster infection in comparison with age-matched immunocompetent patients.[36] In a similar vein, older patients with IBD are at increased risk of developing herpes zoster infection, with the risk of infection higher among patients with IBD than non-IBD individuals in every decade of life (**Fig. 2**). Furthermore, increased rates of disseminated disease and mortality have been demonstrated among those with IBD.

The herpes zoster vaccine is a live attenuated virus vaccine which, like other live vaccines, is generally contraindicated in patients on immunosuppressive medications. However, guidelines by the Advisory Committee on Immunization Practices (ACIP) suggest that the vaccine can be given to patients receiving "low-dose immunosuppression," which includes steroid therapy (<20 mg/d), azathioprine (<3 mg/kg/d), 6-mercaptopurine (1.5 mg/kg/d), and methotrexate (<0.4 mg/kg weekly); these are doses that might commonly be used in IBD.[37] These guidelines advise against administration of the vaccine in the setting of anti-TNF therapy, and suggest temporary discontinuation of these agents for at least 1 month if vaccination is desired. However, subsequently published evidence demonstrates that herpes zoster vaccine is safe when administered to older adults on anti-TNF therapies, and is effective in reducing infection rates in comparison with nonvaccinated controls,[38] suggesting that herpes zoster vaccination should be considered on a case-by-case basis for all patients with IBD who are older than 60 years, even if patients are on thiopurines, and even among patients on anti-TNF agents.

Summary of Vaccine Recommendations for Elderly Patients with IBD

Recommendations for vaccinations in adults with IBD do not significantly differ from those for younger patients, with a few notable exceptions. Influenza vaccination with

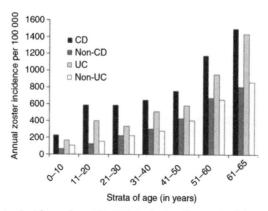

Fig. 2. Annual zoster incidence (per 100,000) in Crohn disease (CD) (n = 50,932) compared with non-CD populations (n = 203,728), and ulcerative colitis (UC) (n = 56,403) compared with non-UC populations (n = 225,612), within 10-year strata of age. (*From* Long MD, Martin C, Sandler RS, et al. Increased risk of herpes zoster among 108 604 patients with inflammatory bowel disease. Aliment Pharmacol Ther 2013;37(4):420–9; with permission.)

the inactivated vaccine should be administered annually. Current recommendations do not yet advocate for a higher-dose vaccine, although it may be more protective and potentially of benefit to those with altered immunity who are at risk for blunted immune responses. Pneumococcal vaccination with PSV23 should be administered at the age of 65 years, even if an individual has received prior vaccination, provided that at least 5 years have elapsed since the previous dose. Other vaccines (hepatitis A, hepatitis B, meningococcus) can be given if and when indicated, as per usual adult guidelines. However, special consideration should be given for the herpes zoster vaccine, which is currently recommended for all adults aged 60 or older.

SUMMARY

The percentage of the United States population older than 60 years is rapidly increasing, as the "baby boomer" generation enters its "golden years." Aging is associated with an increasing number of comorbidities, potential drug interactions, a decline in immune-system function, and a weaker response to vaccinations. Elderly patients with chronic gastrointestinal diseases such as viral hepatitis, autoimmune hepatitis, cirrhosis, and IBD suffer from increased rates of vaccine-preventable infections and increased morbidity and mortality. Immunosuppressive therapies for autoimmune conditions such as IBD and autoimmune hepatitis may decrease the body's immunologic response to vaccinations, suggesting a need to develop strategies to monitor and revaccinate when titers are inadequate. These strategies might include higher initial vaccination doses, booster doses, using antibody titers to guide vaccination practices, and conjugated or adjuvanted vaccines. More studies are urgently needed to further clarify the optimal preventive strategies required to reduce the risks of preventable infections in this susceptible population.

CLINICAL VIGNETTE ANSWERS
Case 1

A 74-year-old man with mildly elevated liver enzymes undergoes a workup and is found to have hepatitis C cirrhosis. What vaccinations should be considered?

He should receive the hepatitis A and B vaccines as soon as possible. He should also receive annual (inactivated) influenza vaccination, Tdap if not up to date, and the herpes zoster vaccine. He should also receive the pneumococcus (PSV23) vaccine; if he already received it after the age of 65 he should receive a second (booster) dose, provided that at least 5 years have elapsed since the initial dose.

Case 2

A 66-year-old practicing physician with ulcerative colitis on azathioprine inquires about what vaccines she should receive. What vaccinations should be considered?

She should receive annual (inactivated) influenza vaccination. She should also receive Tdap, hepatitis A, and hepatitis B as per routine guidelines as a health care professional. Vaccination against herpes zoster should also be considered, and can be administered even if on azathioprine as per ACIP recommendations.

REFERENCES

1. Lutz W, Sanderson W, Scherbov S. Doubling of world population unlikely. Nature 1997;387:803–5.

2. Centers for Disease Control and Prevention. Vaccines & preventable diseases. 2009. Available at: www.cdc.gov/vaccines/vpd-vac/. Accessed August 30, 2013.

3. Grubeck-Loebenstein B, Wick G. The aging of the immune system. Adv Immunol 2002;80:243–84 [Systematic reviews and meta-analysis].

4. Montecino-Rodriguez E, Berent-Maoz B, Dorshkind K. Causes, consequences, and reversal of immune system aging. J Clin Invest 2013;123(3):958–65.

5. Pereira LF, de Souza AP, Borges TJ, et al. Impaired in vivo CD4+ T cell expansion and differentiation in aged mice is not solely due to T cell defects: decreased stimulation by aged dendritic cells. Mech Ageing Dev 2011;132(4):187–94.

6. Moro-García MA, Alonso-Arias R, López-Larrea C. Molecular mechanisms involved in the aging of the T-cell immune response. Curr Genomics 2012;13:589–602.

7. Weinberger B, Herndler-Brandstetter D, Schwanninger A, et al. Biology of immune responses to vaccines in elderly persons. Clin Infect Dis 2008;46: 1078–84 [Systematic reviews and meta-analysis].

8. Goodwin K, Viboud C, Simonsen L. Antibody response to influenza vaccination in the elderly: a quantitative review. Vaccine 2006;24:1159–69 [Systematic reviews and meta-analysis].

9. Hainz U, Jenewein B, Asch E, et al. Insufficient protection for healthy elderly adults by tetanus and TBE vaccines. Vaccine 2005;23:3232–5.

10. D'Acremont V, Herzog C, Genton B. Immunogenicity and safety of a virosomal hepatitis A vaccine (Epaxal ®) in the elderly. J Travel Med 2006;13:78–83.

11. Artz AS, Ershler WB, Longo DL. Pneumococcal vaccination and revaccination of older adults. Clin Microbiol Rev 2003;16:308–18 [Systematic reviews and meta-analysis].

12. Khromava AY, Eidex RB, Weld LH, et al. Yellow fever vaccine: an updated assessment of advanced age as a risk factor for serious adverse events. Vaccine 2005; 23:3256–63.

13. Wolters B, Junge U, Dziuba S, et al. Immunogenicity of combined hepatitis A and B vaccine in elderly persons. Vaccine 2003;21:3623–8.

14. Oxman MN, Levin MJ, Johnson GR, et al. A vaccine to prevent herpes zoster and postherpetic neuralgia in older adults. N Engl J Med 2005;352:2271–84.

15. Dorrington MG, Bowdish DM. Immunosenescence and novel vaccination strategies for the elderly. Front Immunol 2013;4:1–10 [Systematic reviews and meta-analysis].

16. Jackson LA, Janoff EN. Pneumococcal vaccination of elderly adults: new paradigms for protection. Clin Infect Dis 2008;47(10):1328–38.

17. Sprenger MJ, Mulder PG, Beyer WE, et al. Impact of influenza on mortality in relation to age and underlying disease, 1967-1989. Int J Epidemiol 1993; 22(2):334.

18. Duchini A, Viernes ME, Nyberg LM, et al. Hepatic decompensation in patients with cirrhosis during infection with influenza A. Arch Intern Med 2000;160(1):113.

19. Chen WH, Kozlovsky BF, Effros RB, et al. Vaccination in the elderly: an immunological perspective. Trends Immunol 2009;30:351–9 [Systematic reviews and meta-analysis].

20. Heidelbaugh JJ, Bruderly M. Cirrhosis and chronic liver failure: part I. Diagnosis and evaluation. Am Fam Physician 2006;74:756.

21. Ghany MG, Strader DB, Thomas DL, et al. Diagnosis, management, and treatment of hepatitis C: an update. Hepatology 2009;49:1335–418.

22. Smith BD, Morgan RL, Beckett GA, et al. Recommendations for the identification of chronic hepatitis C virus infection among persons born during 1945–1965. MMWR Recomm Rep 2012;61(RR-4):1–32.

23. Pramoolsinsap C, Poovorawan Y, Hirsch P, et al. Acute, hepatitis-A super-infection in HBV carriers, or chronic liver disease related to HBV or HCV. Ann Trop Med Parasitol 1999;93(7):745.
24. Sagnelli E, Coppola N, Messina V, et al. HBV superinfection in hepatitis C virus chronic carriers, viral interaction, and clinical course. Hepatology 2002;36(5):1285.
25. Immunization action coalition: vaccination for adults with hepatitis C infection. Available at: http://www.immunize.org/catg.d/p4042.pdf. Accessed August 31, 2013.
26. Krawitt EL. Autoimmune hepatitis. N Engl J Med 2006;354(1):54 [Systematic reviews and meta-analysis].
27. Manns MP, Czaja AJ, Gorham JD, et al. Management of autoimmune hepatitis. Hepatology 2010;51(6):2193–213.
28. Dezfoli S, Melmed GY. Vaccination issues in patients with inflammatory bowel disease receiving immunosuppression. Gastroenterol Hepatol 2012;8:504–12 [Systematic reviews and meta-analysis].
29. Al-Chalabi T, Boccato S, Portmann BC, et al. Autoimmune hepatitis(AIH) in the elderly: a systematic retrospective analysis of a large group of consecutive patients with definite AIH followed at a tertiary referral centre. J Hepatol 2006; 45(4):575–83.
30. Leber B, Spindelboeck W, Stadlbauer V. Infectious complication of acute and chronic liver disease. Semin Respir Crit Care Med 2012;33:80–95.
31. Taneja SK, Dhiman RK. Prevention and management of bacterial infections in cirrhosis. Int J Hepatol 2011;2011:784540.
32. Garcia-Tsao G, Wiest R. Gut microflora in the pathogenesis of the complications of cirrhosis. Best Pract Res Clin Gastroenterol 2004;18:353–72.
33. Pilotto A, Addante F, D'Onofrio G, et al. The comprehensive geriatric assessment and the multidimensional approach: a new look at the older patient with gastroenterological disorders. Gastroenterology 2009;23(6):829–37.
34. Melmed GY, Agarwal N, Frenck RW, et al. Immunosuppression impairs response to pneumococcal polysaccharide vaccination in patients with inflammatory bowel disease. Am J Gastroenterol 2010;105:148–51.
35. Wasan SK, Baker SE, Skolnik PR, et al. A practical guide to vaccinating the inflammatory bowel disease patient. Am J Gastroenterol 2010;105:1231–8.
36. Long MD, Martin C, Sandler RS, et al. Increased risk of herpes zoster among 108 604 patients with inflammatory bowel disease. Aliment Pharmacol Ther 2013; 37(4):420–9.
37. Harpaz R, Ortega-Sanchez IR, Seward JF, Advisory Committee on Immunization Practices (ACIP) Centers for Disease Control and Prevention (CDC). Prevention of herpes zoster: recommendations of the Advisory Committee on Immunization Practices (ACIP). MMWR Recomm Rep 2008;57:1–30 [Systematic reviews and meta-analysis].
38. Zhang J, Xie F, Delzell E, et al. Association between vaccination for herpes zoster and risk of herpes zoster infection among older patients with selected immune-mediated diseases. JAMA 2012;308(1):43–9.

Reflux and Acid Peptic Diseases in the Elderly

Amir Soumekh, MD[a], Felice H. Schnoll-Sussman, MD[a],
Philip O. Katz, MD[b],*

KEYWORDS

- Gastroesophageal reflux disease • Heartburn • Erosive esophagitis
- Proton-pump inhibitor • Barrett esophagus • Elderly • Geriatric

KEY POINTS

- Gastroesophageal reflux disease (GERD) is common in the elderly.
- Among older patients, GERD may be asymptomatic or may present with atypical or extra-esophageal symptoms, such as cough, voice changes, asthma, dyspepsia, epigastric pain, nausea, bloating, and belching, making the diagnosis of GERD difficult in this patient population.
- Severe disease and complications of GERD such as erosive esophagitis, Barrett esophagus, and esophageal cancer appear to occur at higher rates in geriatric patients than in younger patients.
- Among elderly patients, earlier endoscopic evaluation and more aggressive medical therapy for GERD may be warranted.

INTRODUCTION

Gastroesophageal reflux disease (GERD) is defined as the symptoms or complications resulting from the reflux of gastric contents into the esophagus, oropharynx, naso-pharynx, larynx, or lung.[1,2] GERD can be symptomatically graded by the frequency and severity of symptoms and its effect on the patient's quality of life.[2,3] Reflux disease is common in the general population, and is a frequent reason for patients to seek medical care. Elderly patients with GERD and their providers face a unique set of challenges in the diagnosis, monitoring, and treatment of their disease as well as its complications.

The authors have no relevant financial relationships to disclose.
[a] Division of Gastroenterology and Hepatology, Department of Medicine, Weill Cornell Medical College, 1305 York Avenue, 4th Floor, New York, NY 10021, USA; [b] Division of Gastroenterology, Albert Einstein Medical Center, Thomas Jefferson University, 5401 Old York Road, Klein Professional Building, Suite 363, Philadelphia, PA 19141, USA
* Corresponding author.
E-mail address: katzp@einstein.edu

EPIDEMIOLOGY

GERD is the most commonly seen upper gastrointestinal (GI) condition in primary care. In the United States, it is estimated that approximately one-half of adults experience heartburn at least once a month; 20% report symptoms on a weekly basis, and more than 15 million Americans experience heartburn every day.[1,4–6] The prevalence and associated use of proton-pump inhibitors (PPIs) for the treatment of GERD appears to be rising.[3,7] Recent epidemiologic data suggest that in subjects 65 years and older, rates of GI disorders are particularly high, and are estimated to be the third most common cause of visits to primary care physicians.[8,9] Of these GI disorders, GERD is widely believed to increase with age, as does the propensity for more serious disease, including severe esophagitis, peptic stricture, Barrett esophagus, and esophageal cancer.[10,11]

Esophageal manometry with 24-hour esophageal pH studies shows that frequency and duration of esophageal acid exposure increases with age.[12,13] In a population-based study, the incidence of GERD was significantly higher in the elderly. In patients aged 60 to 69 years the annual incidence was 0.92% in men and 0.68% in women, whereas in the 20- to 29-year age group it was 0.40% in men and 0.35% in women.[14] Endoscopic studies also show increased reflux and more severe esophagitis in elderly patients. In a large study of almost 12,000 patients with reflux esophagitis, severe reflux esophagitis became more prevalent with age, from 12% of patients younger than 21 years to 37% in those older than 70.[15] This finding was corroborated by a retrospective study showing a similar increase in the prevalence of severe esophagitis with increasing age.[16] However, a recent systematic review found no clear evidence that the prevalence of symptom-defined GERD increases with age.[17] This discordance may be due to reduced symptoms of existing GERD in the elderly, at least in part attributable to decreased pain perception.[18] There are data showing that the prevalence of symptoms from GERD appears stable or even decreases with age, despite the aforementioned data showing a rising prevalence of the disease itself.[16] When symptoms do occur, the severity of symptoms and the impairment of quality of life from GERD appear to increase with age; in one study, 6.6% of patients in their forties described their heartburn and/or regurgitation as sufficiently severe to impair lifestyle, compared with 17% of patients in their seventies.[19]

Multiple potential factors aggravate GERD in the elderly, including medications known to reduce lower esophageal sphincter (LES) tone, higher frequency of hiatal hernia, impaired esophageal peristalsis, and decreased saliva volume and bicarbonate concentration.[12,20–24] Limitations in the activities of daily living, common among the elderly, appear to be a significant independent risk factor for reflux.[25] Recently, even postural changes seen in the elderly secondary to changes in bone mineral density and paraspinal muscle strength have been associated with an increased risk of GERD.[26] A final likely reason for the increased severity of GERD in older individuals is the cumulative acid injury over time to the esophageal mucosa and the oropharynx.[27,28]

SYMPTOMS

Heartburn is the hallmark symptom of GERD, characterized by a retrosternal "burning" feeling rising from the stomach or lower chest and radiating toward the neck, throat, and occasionally the back.[2] It often occurs postprandially, particularly after large meals or certain "trigger" foods such as spicy or acidic foods, citrus products, fats, caffeine, and alcohol.[29] Regurgitation of acidic fluids is highly suggestive of GERD, especially if exacerbated by the supine position and bending over. GERD is usually diagnosed symptomatically on the basis of heartburn occurring 2 or more times a week, although less frequent symptoms may still indicate the disease.[2]

As already noted, there are conflicting data on the frequency and severity of symptoms of GERD in the elderly. Some studies show that older patients are less likely than younger patients to report frequent symptoms of GERD.[16–18,30,31] Older patients frequently present with atypical or extraesophageal manifestations of GERD.[32,33] Atypical symptoms include dyspepsia, epigastric pain, nausea, bloating, and belching, which may indicate GERD but may overlap with other conditions.[1] Extraesophageal manifestations of reflux include asthma, chronic cough, and laryngitis.[1,34–36] In this setting, GERD symptoms must be differentiated from those related to gastric disorders (eg, peptic ulcer disease), infectious and motor disorders of the esophagus, and hepatobiliary disorders.[37] These atypical and extraesophageal symptoms may be even more common than typical symptoms in the geriatric population, and may be responsible for a delay in diagnosis in this age group.[11,25,38] Thus, GERD should be suspected in elderly patients with atypical angina, pulmonary disorders that are difficult to manage, voice changes, or intractable hoarseness once cardiopulmonary factors are excluded.

Many elderly patients first present with alarm symptoms such as anemia, dysphagia, odynophagia, or vomiting, because of long-standing disease with minimal traditional symptoms.[37] Dysphagia is common in adults with GERD,[39] usually occurring in the setting of long-standing heartburn with slowly progressive dysphagia for solids, rarely progressing to liquids. Because appetite is unchanged weight loss is typically absent, a clinical clue that may distinguish this benign form of dysphagia from that associated with malignancy.[37] Odynophagia (pain on swallowing) may be seen with severe ulcerative esophagitis, although its presence should raise the suspicion of an alternative cause of esophagitis (eg, infection-induced or drug-induced).

DIAGNOSIS

In younger patients, current practice guidelines allow for a presumptive diagnosis of GERD in the setting of typical symptoms, and recommend initial treatment with an empiric trial of acid-suppression therapy.[1] Diagnostic testing, including upper endoscopy, is reserved for those patients presenting with alarm symptoms, symptoms resistant to medical therapy, or chronic relapsing symptoms. A trial of PPIs is recognized as the first-line test of choice in young patients presenting with traditional or atypical symptoms. Empiric treatment with PPI, as a test for GERD, has sensitivity of 68% to 83%.[40,41] In the typical clinical setting, a PPI trial is preferred because it is universally available, easy to perform, noninvasive, and inexpensive. Moreover, it avoids further invasive or complicated testing in patients who respond.

To date, no guidelines exist on the optimal method of diagnosis of GERD in the elderly. These patients may benefit from early endoscopy rather than an empiric PPI trial, as geriatric patients may have vague or mild symptoms despite the presence of severe esophagitis and even complications of GERD.[25,38] For the same reasons, older patients with atypical symptoms, extraesophageal symptoms, or a history of GERD should be considered for endoscopy. Early endoscopy may detect the presence of erosive esophagitis and allow a better definition of GERD complications, especially strictures, Barrett esophagus, and, possibly, early cancer. Equally important, diagnostic testing may help rule out gastroesophageal reflux or identify an unrelated cause of symptoms, obviating antisecretory therapy and its associated costs and risks. Other diagnostic approaches and tests used to examine elderly patients with GERD are similar to those used in younger adults. Barium esophagography is helpful in suspected oropharyngeal dysphagia or esophageal dysmotility; however, true esophageal dysphagia calls for endoscopy to look for Schatzki rings, peptic strictures, and Barrett esophagus.[42] Esophageal pH and pH-impedance monitoring is helpful to diagnose GERD in several settings. Patients with typical GERD symptoms who do not respond to PPI therapy or who do not have esophagitis on upper endoscopy may benefit from such testing to confirm acid reflux or identify weakly acidic or nonacid reflux as the cause of their symptoms. There are few data on such testing specifically in elderly subjects, as well as some evidence that normative values for pH analysis may not apply to the geriatric population.[43,44] However, such testing can identify elderly patients with GERD who have no evidence of reflux esophagitis on endoscopy.[45] In cases where testing is indicated, prolonged pH monitoring for 48, 72, or 96 hours using a wireless pH capsule system may increase the yield of reflux testing in comparison with 24-hour catheter-based monitoring.[46,47] Patients of any age being evaluated for antireflux surgery, including the elderly, require a comprehensive diagnostic workup to confirm definitively the existence of GERD and to rule out an underlying dysmotility. This evaluation should include upper endoscopy, barium esophagogram, pH testing, and manometry.[48]

COMPLICATIONS

Complications of GERD include erosive esophagitis, peptic stricture, and Barrett esophagus (with the associated risk of esophageal adenocarcinoma). Elderly patients with reflux often first present with alarm symptoms (eg, anemia, dysphagia, odynophagia, vomiting, unintentional weight loss) and complications of GERD attributable to long-standing disease without typical symptoms.[37] For example, up to one-third of elderly patients with Barrett esophagus are asymptomatic at presentation.[49] Furthermore, the frequency of GERD complications appear to be significantly higher as patients age, with one series showing a notably higher rate of erosive esophagitis and Barrett esophagus in patients aged 60 years and older when compared with younger individuals (81% vs 47%).[27] As noted earlier, elderly patients with GERD symptoms may benefit from early endoscopy. All patients who are at high risk for Barrett esophagus should be considered for endoscopy regardless of age.[50] Severe erosive esophagitis may obscure underlying Barrett changes, making endoscopic and pathologic diagnosis difficult.[51,52] When severe esophagitis is noted, biopsies should be deferred and endoscopy repeated after an 8-week course of PPI therapy aimed at healing the erosive disease to rule out Barrett esophagus.[1] Early diagnosis and close surveillance of Barrett esophagus is critical, as esophageal adenocarcinoma is seen with greater frequency in patients older than 60. There is a suggestion of higher morbidity and mortality from esophagectomy in comparison with younger patients[53–55] because dysplasia and early-stage malignancy may be more amenable to treatment with endoscopic therapies (including radiofrequency ablation and endoscopic mucosal resection), as in younger patients, with significantly reduced risk compared with surgery.[50,56]

Chronic reflux esophagitis causes a cycle of scarring, healing, and, ultimately, formation of peptic stricture.[57] Strictures, though relatively uncommon in the setting of PPI use, are more frequent in the elderly than in younger patients, possibly related to long-standing asymptomatic GERD.[38,58] Strictures may be asymptomatic (if there is no significant luminal narrowing) or may cause dysphagia. Strictures may be identified on a barium esophagogram or seen on upper endoscopy. Treatment with endoscopic dilatation is associated with a high success rate and a low rate of complications such as esophageal perforation.[57] Aggressive concomitant management of GERD is required, as ongoing reflux is associated with a higher risk of recurrence.[59] Peptic strictures are typically found in the distal esophagus, often contiguous with the gastro-esophageal junction, and may be near areas of erosive esophagitis. Strictures with atypical features or an atypical location should be biopsied to rule out malignancy.

TREATMENT
Goals of GERD Therapy in an Elderly Population

The treatment goals of GERD in the elderly are similar to those in any adult patient, namely to relieve symptoms, promote mucosal healing, manage complications, and maintain remission.[42,60] As the elderly are prone to more severe esophagitis and potentially higher risk of complications, more aggressive therapy may be warranted. Treatment options include pharmacologic and nonpharmacologic therapies that modify diet and lifestyle, raise gastric pH, and increase esophageal clearance. In some cases, surgical and endoscopic therapies may be warranted.

Dietary and Lifestyle Modifications

There is limited evidence for most lifestyle and dietary modifications in the treatment of GERD. However, these changes are considered as first-line management techniques, and are likely to be as effective in the elderly as in younger patients.[1]

Obesity is associated with an increased risk of GERD, and weight gain is associated with increased frequency of reflux symptoms.[61] Moreover, recent studies confirm the efficacy of weight loss, including in the setting of bariatric surgery, in reducing or eliminating reflux symptoms.[62–64] Therefore, weight loss is recommended for GERD patients who are overweight or have had recent weight gain.

Head-of-bed elevation is recommended for patients with nocturnal or supine symptoms. Randomized controlled trials have shown reduced reflux symptoms and esophageal acid exposure with positional changes, and with the use of blocks or foam wedges under the patient's head and chest or underneath the head of the bed.[65–67] Similarly, patients with nighttime symptoms should be instructed to avoid late evening meals, specifically avoiding high-fat meals within 2 to 3 hours before bedtime.[68,69]

Drugs that promote GERD by reducing LES tone or by acidifying gastric contents should be avoided when possible.[70–72] These agents include anticholinergics, benzodiazepines, opiates, nitrates, calcium-channel antagonists, and hormone replacement therapy. Similarly, medications that are known to cause esophageal injury, such as alendronate, gelatin-capsule antibiotics, iron sulfate, potassium tablets, and nonsteroidal anti-inflammatory drugs (NSAIDs), should be administered with caution in older patients with GERD.

Finally, avoidance of food triggers such as chocolate, caffeine, spicy foods, citrus foods, or carbonated beverages is recommended only in patients who can identify an exacerbation in symptoms with specific foods. There is limited evidence that routine avoidance of all of these potential triggers reduces GERD frequency, severity, or complications, so these changes are not routinely recommended.[1,73]

Over-The-Counter Drugs

Antacids, alginic acid, or over-the-counter (OTC) histamine$_2$ receptor antagonists (H$_2$RAs) may be helpful in relieving mild, transient reflux symptoms.

Antacids, typically containing calcium carbonate, magnesium trisilicate, or aluminum hydroxide, work by neutralizing gastric pH and the resulting refluxate rapidly. These agents have a short duration of action (typically 30–60 minutes) and do not provide long-lasting relief of symptoms.[74] Though typically well tolerated, their use can be limited by side effects. Magnesium-containing agents can cause diarrhea and should be used with caution in patients with renal insufficiency because of an associated risk of hypermagnesemia. Significant intake of calcium carbonate is associated with a risk of developing milk-alkali syndrome. Elderly patients may be at increased risk for this syndrome because of frequent concomitant use of medications such as angiotensin-converting enzyme inhibitors, thiazide diuretics, and NSAIDs.[75] Aluminum-based antacids raise serum aluminum levels, which has been associated with a theoretical (unproven) risk for development of Alzheimer disease.[76]

H_2RAs can be helpful in relieving occasional reflux symptoms but usually do not result in the complete healing of erosive esophagitis[1,42,77] The effectiveness of H_2RAs is limited by a relatively short duration of action, the development of tachyphylaxis, and incomplete inhibition of meal-stimulated acid secretion.[78]

Prescription Medications

PPIs provide significantly improved efficacy in controlling reflux symptoms and complications by suppressing gastric acid secretion to a greater degree and for a longer duration than antacids and H_2 blockers.[79] In 43 randomized controlled trials involving more than 7000 patients, erosive esophagitis healed in 84% of patients treated with PPIs, versus 52% of those treated with H_2RAs.[80] Time to healing was also significantly reduced in patients on PPIs.

Several PPIs are currently available in the United States, including esomeprazole, lansoprazole, dexlansoprazole, omeprazole, omeprazole-IR, pantoprazole, and rabeprazole. Omeprazole, omeprazole-IR, and lansoprazole are available as OTC formulations. Esomeprazole should be available in the near future. Regardless of the patient's age, a single dose of any PPI for a standard 8-week course of therapy yields high healing rates of erosive esophagitis, ranging from 73% to 91%.[81]

Elderly patients with GERD have more severe esophagitis, and PPIs may be particularly useful in this patient population.[15,16] Elderly patients may require more acid suppression for esophagitis healing, and PPIs achieve significantly more healing in erosive esophagitis than do H_2RAs.[30,82,83] Following healing of esophagitis and improvement of symptoms, long-term acid-suppression therapy may be required to control GERD symptoms and maintain esophageal healing; up to 90% of elderly patients may relapse within a year if PPIs are discontinued.[83,84] Higher dosing of PPIs is often necessary to achieve and then maintain healing of esophagitis in older adults. In one study, maintenance therapy with pantoprazole, 20 mg daily for 6 months, kept 84% of adults aged up to 88 years (N = 396) in remission, compared with 93% with pantoprazole 40 mg daily.[85] In another study of 103 patients, after 1 year of treatment with lansoprazole, the healing rates were 72% with 15 mg daily and 85% with 30 mg daily.[86] After 12 months of maintenance therapy, the rates of remission from erosive esophagitis observed among 164 patients aged 65 years and older were 79.6% (95% confidence interval [CI] 68.3%–90.9%) and 30.4% (95% CI 18.3%–42.4%) for pantoprazole 20 mg once daily and placebo, respectively (number needed to treat, 2; $P = .0001$). Heartburn, acid regurgitation, and chest pain were significantly associated with the relapse of erosive esophagitis ($P = .0001$).

Pharmacokinetic Considerations and Long-Term Tolerability of PPIs

Some age-related pharmacokinetic effects on the metabolism of PPIs have been reported in the elderly. Klotz[87] compared published pharmacokinetic data for 4 PPIs in young and elderly populations, and found significant increases in half-life and reductions in plasma clearance in elderly patients treated with lansoprazole, omeprazole, or rabeprazole. By contrast, the pharmacokinetics of pantoprazole and esomeprazole seem to be relatively unaffected by age.[88,89] The clinical relevance of these differences in pharmacokinetics is unclear. When comorbidities are involved, the dosage regimen should be tailored to the individual patient, and should take into account concomitant illnesses, therapies, and any organ impairments that may potentially alter the efficacy or tolerability of PPIs.

PPIs appear to be well tolerated with chronic long-term use, although there has been recent concern about long-term side effects such as nutritional deficiencies, infectious complications, and changes in bone mineral density.[90] Common side effects include headaches, nausea, abdominal pain, constipation, flatulence, diarrhea, rash, and dizziness.

A theoretical risk of vitamin B_{12} deficiency with chronic PPI use, resulting from a lack of gastric acid, has not been borne out in the general population. However, case reports and series have shown some association between long-term PPI use and lowered B_{12} levels in the elderly.[91-93] It is not yet clear whether routine serum B_{12} measurements are warranted.

A relationship between antisecretory therapy and infections, specifically pneumonia and enteric infections, has been raised, but the data are mixed. Retrospective cross-sectional data, randomized controlled trials, and meta-analyses have yielded conflicting findings on the association between PPI use and pneumonia.[94] Data on this association specifically within the elderly population have not identified a clear link.[95] However, there is mounting evidence that chronic acid suppression increases the risk of infection by a variety of enteric pathogens, including *Clostridium difficile*.[96] Studies on the risk of *C difficile* infections specifically among elderly PPI users are limited, and have not confirmed such an association.[97]

In vitro and in vivo studies in humans and animals have shown a decrease in calcium absorption and alterations in osteoclast function with PPI use, raising concern for an increased risk of osteoporosis and osteoporotic fractures.[94] No large-scale randomized trials or long-term prospective studies have been performed to assess this risk, and existing studies have shown conflicting results. One large case-control review of more than 15,000 patients older than 50 years with osteoporosis-related fractures did show an association between long-term (>7 years) PPI exposure and fracture risk. However, these data are insufficient to warrant routine bone mineral density screening or pharmacologic prophylaxis for osteoporosis at present.[94] It is reasonable to check serum vitamin D levels and correct for vitamin D deficiency. For PPI users who require calcium supplementation, a soluble form such as calcium citrate is preferred.

Antireflux Surgery

Surgical treatment of GERD is generally reserved for selected patients in whom the diagnosis is confirmed and for whom lifestyle changes and antisecretory therapy alone do not resolve symptoms. Studies on antireflux surgery in the elderly show high response rates in both short-term and long-term follow-up.[98-100] Although there is often a perception that older patients may not be able to tolerate a surgical procedure such as a Nissen fundoplication, studies with both open and laparoscopic Nissen fundoplication have found no increase in the mortality, morbidity, or hospital stay in patients older than 60 years in comparison with their younger counterparts.[101-103]

Careful preoperative evaluation is important in all patients considered for antireflux surgery, especially the elderly. Endoscopy needs to be performed to exclude Barrett esophagus with dysplasia or early cancer. Esophageal manometry may help identify patients with weak esophageal peristalsis before surgery, to avoid postoperative dysphagia or bloating. Esophageal 24-hour pH monitoring is recommended in symptomatic patients without esophagitis to confirm the diagnosis, and in patients with intractable esophagitis to exclude drug-induced esophagitis. Finally, selected patients with nausea, vomiting, or severe abdominal bloating may need gastric-emptying studies to exclude gastroparesis.

SUMMARY

Managing GERD in geriatric patients can be complex. Elderly patients often present to the clinician late or with complications, and their diagnosis (and treatment) is often delayed, because of a lack of typical reflux symptoms, a higher rate of atypical and extraesophageal symptoms, and a baseline tendency toward more severe disease. Early endoscopy should be considered in elderly patients with GERD, regardless of symptom severity.

Overall, the treatment of acid reflux in the elderly is similar to that used in younger adults. Although studies on this age group are limited, there is a need for more aggressive workup and treatment in this population because of the increased severity of disease and the increased rate of complications associated with GERD. The success of medical and surgical therapy is high in older patients, although treatments must be selected carefully and patients monitored for side effects.

REFERENCES

1. Katz PO, Gerson LB, Vela MF. Guidelines for the diagnosis and management of gastroesophageal reflux disease. Am J Gastroenterol 2013;108(3):308–28 [quiz: 329].
2. Vakil N, van Zanten SV, Kahrilas P, et al. The Montreal definition and classification of gastroesophageal reflux disease: a global evidence-based consensus. Am J Gastroenterol 2006;101(8):1900–20 [quiz: 1943].
3. El-Serag HB, Sweet S, Winchester CC, et al. Update on the epidemiology of gastro-oesophageal reflux disease: a systematic review. Gut 2013;1–10.
4. Johanson JF. Epidemiology of esophageal and supraesophageal reflux injuries. Am J Med 2000;108(Suppl 4a):99S–103S.
5. Sobieraj DM, Coleman SM, Coleman CI. US prevalence of upper gastrointestinal symptoms: a systematic literature review. Am J Manag Care 2011;17(11):e449–58.
6. Locke GR 3rd, Talley NJ, Fett SL, et al. Prevalence and clinical spectrum of gastroesophageal reflux: a population-based study in Olmsted County, Minnesota. Gastroenterology 1997;112(5):1448–56.
7. Friedenberg FK, Hanlon A, Vanar V, et al. Trends in gastroesophageal reflux disease as measured by the National Ambulatory Medical Care Survey. Dig Dis Sci 2010;55(7):1911–7.
8. Friedman LS. Gastrointestinal disorders in the elderly. Gastroenterol Clin North Am 1990;19(2):227–457.
9. Crane SJ, Talley NJ. Chronic gastrointestinal symptoms in the elderly. Clin Geriatr Med 2007;23(4):721–34, v.
10. el-Serag HB, Sonnenberg A. Associations between different forms of gastro-oesophageal reflux disease. Gut 1997;41(5):594–9.
11. Mold JW, Reed LE, Davis AB, et al. Prevalence of gastroesophageal reflux in elderly patients in a primary care setting. Am J Gastroenterol 1991;86(8):965–70.
12. Lee J, Anggiansah A, Anggiansah R, et al. Effects of age on the gastroesophageal junction, esophageal motility, and reflux disease. Clin Gastroenterol Hepatol 2007;5(12):1392–8.
13. Ter RB, Johnston BT, Castell DO. Influence of age and gender on gastroesophageal reflux in symptomatic patients. Dis Esophagus 1998;11(2):106–8.

14. Ruigomez A, García Rodríguez LA, Wallander MA, et al. Natural history of gastro-oesophageal reflux disease diagnosed in general practice. Aliment Pharmacol Ther 2004;20(7):751–60.

15. Johnson DA, Fennerty MB. Heartburn severity underestimates erosive esophagitis severity in elderly patients with gastroesophageal reflux disease. Gastroenterology 2004;126(3):660–4.

16. Pilotto A, Franceschi M, Leandro G, et al. Clinical features of reflux esophagitis in older people: a study of 840 consecutive patients. J Am Geriatr Soc 2006; 54(10):1537–42.

17. Becher A, Dent J. Systematic review: ageing and gastro-oesophageal reflux disease symptoms, oesophageal function and reflux oesophagitis. Aliment Pharmacol Ther 2011;33(4):442–54.

18. Mold JW, Rankin RA. Symptomatic gastroesophageal reflux in the elderly. J Am Geriatr Soc 1987;35(7):649–59.

19. Diaz-Rubio M, Moreno-Elola-Olaso C, Rey E, et al. Symptoms of gastro-oesophageal reflux: prevalence, severity, duration and associated factors in a Spanish population. Aliment Pharmacol Ther 2004;19(1):95–105.

20. Stanghellini V. Three-month prevalence rates of gastrointestinal symptoms and the influence of demographic factors: results from the Domestic/International Gastroenterology Surveillance Study (DIGEST). Scand J Gastroenterol Suppl 1999;231:20–8.

21. Khan TA, Shragge BW, Crispin JS, et al. Esophageal motility in the elderly. Am J Dig Dis 1977;22(12):1049–54.

22. Stilson WL, Sanders I, Gardiner GA, et al. Hiatal hernia and gastroesophageal reflux. A clinicoradiological analysis of more than 1,000 cases. Radiology 1969;93(6):1323–7.

23. Achem AC, Achem SR, Stark ME, et al. Failure of esophageal peristalsis in older patients: association with esophageal acid exposure. Am J Gastroenterol 2003; 98(1):35–9.

24. Richter JE, Castell DO. Gastroesophageal reflux. Pathogenesis, diagnosis, and therapy. Ann Intern Med 1982;97(1):93–103.

25. Pilotto A, Maggi S, Noale M, et al. Association of upper gastrointestinal symptoms with functional and clinical characteristics in elderly. World J Gastroenterol 2011;17(25):3020–6.

26. Imagama S, Hasegawa Y, Wakao N, et al. Influence of lumbar kyphosis and back muscle strength on the symptoms of gastroesophageal reflux disease in middle-aged and elderly people. Eur Spine J 2012;21(11):2149–57.

27. Zhu H, Pace F, Sangaletti O, et al. Gastric acid secretion and pattern of gastro-esophageal reflux in patients with esophagitis and concomitant duodenal ulcer. A multivariate analysis of pathogenetic factors. Scand J Gastroenterol 1993; 28(5):387–92.

28. Kuchel GA, Hof PR. Autonomic nervous system in old age. Interdisciplinary topics in gerontology. Basel (Switzerland), New York: Karger; 2004. p. 137.

29. Dent J, Brun J, Fendrick A, et al. An evidence-based appraisal of reflux disease management—the Genval Workshop Report. Gut 1999;44(Suppl 2):S1–16.

30. Collen MJ, Abdulian JD, Chen YK. Gastroesophageal reflux disease in the elderly: more severe disease that requires aggressive therapy. Am J Gastroenterol 1995;90(7):1053–7.

31. Ferriolli E, Oliveira RB, Matsuda NM, et al. Aging, esophageal motility, and gastroesophageal reflux. J Am Geriatr Soc 1998;46(12):1534–7.

32. Klauser AG, Schindlbeck NE, Muller-Lissner SA. Symptoms in gastro-oesophageal reflux disease. Lancet 1990;335(8683):205–8.
33. Räihä IJ, Impivaara O, Seppälä M, et al. Prevalence and characteristics of symptomatic gastroesophageal reflux disease in the elderly. J Am Geriatr Soc 1992;40(12):1209–11.
34. DeVault KR. Extraesophageal symptoms of GERD. Cleve Clin J Med 2003; 70(Suppl 5):S20–32.
35. Vaezi MF. Extraesophageal manifestations of gastroesophageal reflux disease. Clin Cornerstone 2003;5(4):32–8 [discussion: 39–40].
36. Napierkowski J, Wong RK. Extraesophageal manifestations of GERD. Am J Med Sci 2003;326(5):285–99.
37. el-Serag HB, Sonnenberg A. Comorbid occurrence of laryngeal or pulmonary disease with esophagitis in United States military veterans. Gastroenterology 1997;113(3):755–60.
38. Maekawa T, Kinoshita Y, Okada A, et al. Relationship between severity and symptoms of reflux oesophagitis in elderly patients in Japan. J Gastroenterol Hepatol 1998;13(9):927–30.
39. Jacob P, Kahrilas PJ, Vanagunas A. Peristaltic dysfunction associated with non-obstructive dysphagia in reflux disease. Dig Dis Sci 1990;35(8):939–42.
40. Fass R, Pulliam G, Johnson C, et al. Symptom severity and oesophageal chemo-sensitivity to acid in older and young patients with gastro-oesophageal reflux. Age Ageing 2000;29(2):125–30.
41. Schindlbeck NE, Klauser AG, Voderholzer WA, et al. Empiric therapy for gastro-esophageal reflux disease. Arch Intern Med 1995;155(16):1808–12.
42. Feldman M, Friedman LS, Brandt LJ. Sleisenger & Fordtran's gastrointestinal and liver disease: pathophysiology, diagnosis, management. 8th edition. Philadelphia: Saunders; 2006.
43. Jalal A, Payne HR, Jeyasingham K. The influence of age on gastro-oesophageal reflux: a re-appraisal of the DeMeester scoring system. Eur J Cardiothorac Surg 2000;18(4):411–7.
44. Zerbib F, des Varannes SB, Roman S, et al. Normal values and day-to-day variability of 24-h ambulatory oesophageal impedance-pH monitoring in a Belgian-French cohort of healthy subjects. Aliment Pharmacol Ther 2005;22(10):1011–21.
45. Wu B. Diagnosis of gastroesophageal reflux disease in elderly subjects using 24-hour esophageal pH monitoring. Chin Med J (Engl) 1999;112(4):333–5.
46. Scarpulla G, Camilleri S, Galante P, et al. The impact of prolonged pH measurements on the diagnosis of gastroesophageal reflux disease: 4-day wireless pH studies. Am J Gastroenterol 2007;102(12):2642–7.
47. Chander B, Hanley-Williams N, Deng Y, et al. 24 versus 48-hour bravo pH monitoring. J Clin Gastroenterol 2012;46(3):197–200.
48. Jobe BA, Richter JE, Hoppo T, et al. Preoperative diagnostic workup before anti-reflux surgery: an evidence and experience-based consensus of the esophageal diagnostic advisory panel. J Am Coll Surg 2013;217(4):586–97.
49. Zimmerman J, Shohat V, Tsvang E, et al. Esophagitis is a major cause of upper gastrointestinal hemorrhage in the elderly. Scand J Gastroenterol 1997;32(9): 906–9.
50. American Gastroenterological Association. American Gastroenterological Association medical position statement on the management of Barrett's esophagus. Gastroenterology 2011;140(3):1084–91.
51. Hanna S, Rastogi A, Weston AP, et al. Detection of Barrett's esophagus after endoscopic healing of erosive esophagitis. Am J Gastroenterol 2006;101(7):1416–20.

52. Rodriguez S, Mattek N, Lieberman D, et al. Barrett's esophagus on repeat endoscopy: should we look more than once? Am J Gastroenterol 2008;103(8):1892–7.

53. Pech O, May A, Gossner L, et al. Curative endoscopic therapy in patients with early esophageal squamous-cell carcinoma or high-grade intraepithelial neoplasia. Endoscopy 2007;39(1):30–5.

54. Thomas P, Doddoli C, Neville P, et al. Esophageal cancer resection in the elderly. Eur J Cardiothorac Surg 1996;10(11):941–6.

55. Birkmeyer JD, Siewers AE, Finlayson EV, et al. Hospital volume and surgical mortality in the United States. N Engl J Med 2002;346(15):1128–37.

56. Morganstern B, Anandasabapathy S. GERD and Barrett's esophagus: diagnostic and management strategies in the geriatric population. Geriatrics 2009; 64(7):9–12.

57. Bansal A, Kahrilas PJ. Treatment of GERD complications (Barrett's, peptic stricture) and extra-oesophageal syndromes. Best Pract Res Clin Gastroenterol 2010;24(6):961–8.

58. Ruigómez A, García Rodríguez LA, Wallander MA, et al. Esophageal stricture: incidence, treatment patterns, and recurrence rate. Am J Gastroenterol 2006; 101(12):2685–92.

59. Said A, Brust DJ, Gaumnitz EA, et al. Predictors of early recurrence of benign esophageal strictures. Am J Gastroenterol 2003;98(6):1252–6.

60. Katzka DA, Rustgi AK. Gastroesophageal reflux disease and Barrett's esophagus. Med Clin North Am 2000;84(5):1137–61.

61. Jacobson BC, Somers SC, Fuchs CS, et al. Body-mass index and symptoms of gastroesophageal reflux in women. N Engl J Med 2006;354(22):2340–8.

62. Fraser-Moodie CA, Norton B, Gornall C, et al. Weight loss has an independent beneficial effect on symptoms of gastro-oesophageal reflux in patients who are overweight. Scand J Gastroenterol 1999;34(4):337–40.

63. Singh M, Lee J, Gupta N, et al. Weight loss can lead to resolution of gastroesophageal reflux disease symptoms: a prospective intervention trial. Obesity (Silver Spring) 2013;21(2):284–90.

64. Ness-Jensen E, Lindam A, Lagergren J, et al. Weight loss and reduction in gastroesophageal reflux. A prospective population-based cohort study: the HUNT study. Am J Gastroenterol 2013;108(3):376–82.

65. Stanciu C, Bennett JR. Effects of posture on gastro-oesophageal reflux. Digestion 1977;15(2):104–9.

66. Hamilton JW, Boisen RJ, Yamamoto DT, et al. Sleeping on a wedge diminishes exposure of the esophagus to refluxed acid. Dig Dis Sci 1988;33(5):518–22.

67. Pollmann H, Zillessen E, Pohl J, et al. Effect of elevated head position in bed in therapy of gastroesophageal reflux. Z Gastroenterol 1996;34(Suppl 2):93–9 [in German].

68. Duroux P, Bauerfeind P, Emde C, et al. Early dinner reduces nocturnal gastric acidity. Gut 1989;30(8):1063–7.

69. Orr WC, Harnish MJ. Sleep-related gastro-oesophageal reflux: provocation with a late evening meal and treatment with acid suppression. Aliment Pharmacol Ther 1998;12(10):1033–8.

70. Slyk MP. Pathophysiology and management challenges of GERD in the seniors. Director 2004;12(3):147–53.

71. Richter JE. Gastroesophageal reflux disease in the older patient: presentation, treatment, and complications. Am J Gastroenterol 2000;95(2):368–73.

72. Weinberg DS, Kadish SL. The diagnosis and management of gastroesophageal reflux disease. Med Clin North Am 1996;80(2):411–29.

73. Johnson T, Gerson L, Hershcovici T, et al. Systematic review: the effects of carbonated beverages on gastro-oesophageal reflux disease. Aliment Pharmacol Ther 2010;31(6):607–14.

74. Sontag SJ. The medical management of reflux esophagitis. Role of antacids and acid inhibition. Gastroenterol Clin North Am 1990;19(3):683–712.

75. Patel AM, Goldfarb S. Got calcium? Welcome to the calcium-alkali syndrome. J Am Soc Nephrol 2010;21(9):1440–3.

76. Tomljenovic L. Aluminum and Alzheimer's disease: after a century of controversy, is there a plausible link? J Alzheimers Dis 2011;23(4):567–98.

77. Fennerty MB, Castell D, Fendrick AM, et al. The diagnosis and treatment of gastroesophageal reflux disease in a managed care environment. Suggested disease management guidelines. Arch Intern Med 1996;156(5):477–84.

78. Colin-Jones DG. The role and limitations of H2-receptor antagonists in the treatment of gastro-oesophageal reflux disease. Aliment Pharmacol Ther 1995;9(Suppl 1):9–14.

79. Robinson M, Horn J. Clinical pharmacology of proton pump inhibitors: what the practising physician needs to know. Drugs 2003;63(24):2739–54.

80. Chiba N, De Gara CJ, Wilkinson JM, et al. Speed of healing and symptom relief in grade II to IV gastroesophageal reflux disease: a meta-analysis. Gastroenterology 1997;112(6):1798–810.

81. Edwards SJ, Lind T, Lundell L. Systematic review: proton pump inhibitors (PPIs) for the healing of reflux oesophagitis—a comparison of esomeprazole with other PPIs. Aliment Pharmacol Ther 2006;24(5):743–50.

82. James OF, Parry-Billings KS. Comparison of omeprazole and histamine H2-receptor antagonists in the treatment of elderly and young patients with reflux oesophagitis. Age Ageing 1994;23(2):121–6.

83. Carlsson R, Galmiche JP, Dent J, et al. Prognostic factors influencing relapse of oesophagitis during maintenance therapy with antisecretory drugs: a meta-analysis of long-term omeprazole trials. Aliment Pharmacol Ther 1997;11(3):473–82.

84. Pilotto A, Franceschi M, Leandro G, et al. Long-term clinical outcome of elderly patients with reflux esophagitis: a six-month to three-year follow-up study. Am J Ther 2002;9(4):295–300.

85. Escourrou J, Deprez P, Saggioro A, et al. Maintenance therapy with pantoprazole 20 mg prevents relapse of reflux oesophagitis. Aliment Pharmacol Ther 1999;13(11):1481–91.

86. Hatlebakk JG, Berstad A. Lansoprazole 15 and 30 mg daily in maintaining healing and symptom relief in patients with reflux oesophagitis. Aliment Pharmacol Ther 1997;11(2):365–72.

87. Klotz U. Effect of aging on the pharmacokinetics of gastrointestinal drugs. In: Pilotto A, Malfertheiner P, Holt PR, editors. Aging and the Gastrointestinal Tract, Vol 32. Basel: Karger; 2003. p. 28–39.

88. Huber R, Hartmann M, Bliesath H, et al. Pharmacokinetics of pantoprazole in man. Int J Clin Pharmacol Ther 1996;34(5):185–94.

89. Hasselgren G, Hassan-Alin M, Andersson T, et al. Pharmacokinetic study of esomeprazole in the elderly. Clin Pharmacokinet 2001;40(2):145–50.

90. Klinkenberg-Knol EC, Nelis F, Dent J, et al. Long-term omeprazole treatment in resistant gastroesophageal reflux disease: efficacy, safety, and influence on gastric mucosa. Gastroenterology 2000;118(4):661–9.

91. Dharmarajan TS, Kanagala MR, Murakonda P, et al. Do acid-lowering agents affect vitamin B12 status in older adults? J Am Med Dir Assoc 2008;9(3):162–7.

92. Valuck RJ, Ruscin JM. A case-control study on adverse effects: H2 blocker or proton pump inhibitor use and risk of vitamin B12 deficiency in older adults. J Clin Epidemiol 2004;57(4):422–8.

93. Rozgony NR, Fang C, Kuczmarski MF, et al. Vitamin B(12) deficiency is linked with long-term use of proton pump inhibitors in institutionalized older adults: could a cyanocobalamin nasal spray be beneficial? J Nutr Elder 2010;29(1): 87–99.

94. Sheen E, Triadafilopoulos G. Adverse effects of long-term proton pump inhibitor therapy. Dig Dis Sci 2011;56(4):931–50.

95. Dublin S, Walker RL, Jackson ML, et al. Use of proton pump inhibitors and H2 blockers and risk of pneumonia in older adults: a population-based case-control study. Pharmacoepidemiol Drug Saf 2010;19(8):792–802.

96. Howell MD, Novack V, Grgurich P, et al. Iatrogenic gastric acid suppression and the risk of nosocomial *Clostridium difficile* infection. Arch Intern Med 2010; 170(9):784–90.

97. Lowe DO, Mamdani MM, Kopp A, et al. Proton pump inhibitors and hospitalization for *Clostridium difficile*-associated disease: a population-based study. Clin Infect Dis 2006;43(10):1272–6.

98. Aprea G, Ferronetti A, Canfora A, et al. GERD in elderly patients: surgical treatment with Nissen-Rossetti laparoscopic technique, outcome. BMC Surg 2012; 12(Suppl 1):S4.

99. Wang W, Huang MT, Wei PL, et al. Laparoscopic antireflux surgery for the elderly: a surgical and quality-of-life study. Surg Today 2008;38(4):305–10.

100. Khajanchee YS, Urbach DR, Butler N, et al. Laparoscopic antireflux surgery in the elderly. Surg Endosc 2002;16(1):25–30.

101. Allen R, Rappaport W, Hixson L, et al. Referral patterns and the results of antireflux operations in patients more than sixty years of age. Surg Gynecol Obstet 1991;173(5):359–62.

102. Tedesco P, Lobo E, Fisichella PM, et al. Laparoscopic fundoplication in elderly patients with gastroesophageal reflux disease. Arch Surg 2006;141(3):289–92 [discussion: 292].

103. Kamolz T, Bammer T, Granderath FA, et al. Quality of life and surgical outcome after laparoscopic antireflux surgery in the elderly gastroesophageal reflux disease patient. Scand J Gastroenterol 2001;36(2):116–20.

Dysphagia in the Elderly

Abraham Khan, MD[a], Richard Carmona, BA[b],
Morris Traube, MD, JD[a],*

KEYWORDS

- Dysphagia • Oropharyngeal • Esophageal • Swallowing • Motility

KEY POINTS

- Dysphagia, or difficulty swallowing, is a common problem in the elderly and can cause malnutrition and significant morbidity.
- Key findings on clinical history and physical examination can suggest whether the patient has either predominantly oropharyngeal or esophageal dysphagia and guide the appropriate workup and treatment of these patients.
- The most common causes of oropharyngeal dysphagia are of neurologic origin and can be managed in conjunction with a clinical swallow specialist.
- Esophageal dysphagia may result from structural or functional disorders, and a video barium esophagram is a good initial test in the workup of these patients. Often a gastroenterologist will be consulted for evaluation, endoscopy, or manometry, followed by appropriate treatment.

INTRODUCTION

Dysphagia, or difficulty swallowing, is a common problem in the elderly. For example, nearly 50% of all patients residing in nursing homes suffer from a swallowing disorder.[1] One study found that 63% of elderly patients who denied any history of swallowing difficulties had abnormal swallowing parameters on radiologic swallow studies.[2]

The problem will certainly become more widespread. From 2010 to 2030, the elderly population is expected to increase from 39 million to 69 million Americans.[3] In 2050, elderly Americans, defined as those at least 65 years old, are expected to make up 20% of the total population, a substantial increase from 13% in 2010.[4] In addition to the discomfort that patients have from dysphagia, the complications associated with swallowing difficulty are substantial. Elderly patients with dysphagia have a significantly elevated risk of malnutrition and aspiration pneumonia. This risk is particularly

[a] Division of Gastroenterology, Department of Medicine and Center for Esophageal Disease, NYU School of Medicine, 530 First Avenue, SKR 9N, New York, NY 10016, USA; [b] NYU School of Medicine, 550 First Avenue, New York, NY 10016, USA
* Corresponding author.
E-mail address: Morris.Traube@nyumc.org

true in the subpopulation with oropharyngeal dysphagia of neurologic origin, that is, cerebrovascular disease, brain injury, or neurodegenerative disease.

A study using the Subjective Global Assessment (SGA) to assess nutritional status found that 16% of patients with dysphagia related to nonprogressive brain disorders had concomitant malnutrition, whereas malnutrition was noted in 22% of patients whose dysphagia stemmed from neurodegenerative disease.[5] Elderly patients with malnutrition resulting from dysphagia show increased morbidity and mortality from several factors, including, but not limited to, a lowered immune response, decreased ability to recover from illness and heal wounds, and weakened respiratory drive/muscle strength.[6,7] Because of the likelihood of choking and aspirating with a swallowing disorder, which can aid in bacterial colonization, aspiration pneumonia is also common in patients with dysphagia. Up to 50% of patients with oropharyngeal dysphagia in nursing homes have aspiration pneumonia within 1 year, and the mortality rate approaches 45%.[5]

ANATOMY AND PHYSIOLOGY OF SWALLOWING

Before reviewing the specific swallowing disorders and the relevant approach to diagnosis, a basic understanding of the anatomy and physiology of swallowing is essential.[8] Typically, the process of swallowing is broken down into 3 primary phases: oral, pharyngeal, and esophageal. The oral phase, the only voluntary phase of swallowing, is often divided again into 2 subphases: the preparatory and transport phases.

During the oral preparatory phase, food enters into the oral cavity to be chewed and formed into an appropriate bolus for swallowing. This phase is dependent on voluntary action of chewing and swallowing the meal for nutrition. The coordinated manipulation and mastication of the food depends on several facial muscles and their cranial nerve signals, whereas chemoreceptors and mechanoreceptors are responsible for the stimulation of salivary glands. When the food has been adequately manipulated by means of mastication and salivary coating, the oral transport phase occurs. During this phase, the tongue moves the bolus posteriorly toward the oropharynx for swallowing.

During the pharyngeal phase, the velopharyngeal muscles mediate the closure of the nasopharynx to avoid nasal regurgitation. Preventing food from entering into the airway is one of the most important aspects of swallowing and requires the coordinated effort of the epiglottis, the vocal cords, and the larynx. The first step of this process is the closure of the true vocal cords, which is the most reliable protection against aspiration. This is followed by closure of the false vocal cords and superior displacement of the larynx. The superior and anterior placement of the larynx inverts the epiglottis so that it can further protect against aspiration. The other major function of the retroverted epiglottis is to route the bolus to the pyriform sinuses located on opposite sides of the pharynx. From the pyriform sinuses, the superior, middle, and inferior constrictor muscles contract respectively and are responsible for pharyngeal peristalsis. Mechanoreceptors are then continuously stimulated to promote the contraction of pharyngeal muscles until the bolus has completely passed into the esophagus. The pharyngeal phase of swallowing terminates when the bolus passes through the upper esophageal sphincter (UES), which is composed mostly of the cricopharyngeus muscle and fibers from the inferior pharyngeal constrictor.

After the bolus passes the UES, the esophageal phase of swallowing begins, and is entirely under involuntary control. The esophagus has 2 muscle layers, an inner circular muscle layer and an outer longitudinal muscle layer. Both central and peripheral neuromuscular control are necessary to pass the bolus from the striated muscle portion of the upper esophagus to the smooth muscle portion of the more distal esophagus and ultimately through the smooth muscle lower esophageal sphincter

(LES). The food bolus normally passes through the esophagus and into the stomach in 8 to 10 seconds. This coordinated series of contractions is referred to as *esophageal peristalsis*. Once the swallow is initiated, the LES relaxes. This relaxation is mediated by the vagus nerve and persists until the food bolus enters the stomach.[9]

PATHOPHYSIOLOGY OF DEGLUTITION IN THE ELDERLY

Two major types of dysphagia are used to describe abnormal swallowing. Patients can have oropharyngeal dysphagia, esophageal dysphagia, or a combination of both. Oropharyngeal dysphagia results from dysfunction in the swallowing process before food enters into the esophagus. Several changes in the elderly may predispose to dysphagia. Loss of jaw strength, salivary production, and dentition, as well as increased connective and fatty tissue in the tongue can affect the oral phase of swallowing.[10,11] However, typically, age-related changes to this phase of swallowing do not result in dysphagia. In the pharyngeal phase, the threshold needed for laryngeal elevation is increased and the elevation is less marked. After the age of 60, pharyngeal swallowing is significantly longer, sometimes requires multiple swallows per bolus, and can greatly increase the risk of aspiration.[12] The initiation of the esophageal phase can also be delayed in the elderly, resulting from a loss of UES elasticity or compliance.[11]

Along with these age-related changes, some neurologic disorders are much more common in the elderly and contribute to the increased prevalence of dysphagia. These disorders include transient ischemic attacks, strokes, and neurodegenerative diseases, such as Parkinson's disease. Other causes of dysphagia that are increased in the elderly include Zenker's diverticulum, achalasia, and esophageal tumors. These disorders are discussed below.

APPROACH TO DIAGNOSIS
History and Physical Examination

Taking a careful history and performing a physical examination is of extreme importance and is the first step in the diagnosis of dysphagia (**Box 1**). Three common related symptoms of dysphagia in the elderly include eating meals more slowly; choking, coughing, or throat-clearing either during or after meals; and feeling as if food is stuck

---

Box 1
Dysphagia: key associated findings

Historical Findings

- Choking, coughing, or throat clearing during or after meals
- Food stuck in throat or mid-chest
- Frequent pulmonary infections
- Weight loss, change in diet or consistency of food
- Neurologic changes

Physical Examination Findings

- Loss of dentition
- Abnormal lip closure or tongue range of motion
- Vocal changes
- Neurologic deficits

in the throat.[13] The patient should also be asked about any weight loss, general changes in diet or consistency of food, or neurologic changes. A history of smoking and alcohol abuse should raise concern of malignancy in both oropharyngeal and esophageal dysphagia.[1]

Certainly, dysphagia can be of acute onset as seen in a stroke; however, more often, dysphagia is of slow onset and only slowly progressive. Because of this insidious nature, patients often change the consistency of their food to avoid symptoms. Detail of the food consistencies that cause difficulty may also help discover the cause of dysphagia. Often, patients who struggle to swallow more with solid foods suffer from an obstruction, such as a stricture, ring, or web, whereas those who struggle with liquids are more likely to have dysphagia of neurologic origin. Furthermore, a history of frequent pulmonary infections may suggest that the patient is suffering from dysphagia and recurrent aspiration.

On physical examination, the oral cavity should be examined for loss of dentition, abnormal lip closure and strength of closure, and tongue range of motion. Voice quality should also be assessed, with careful attention paid to either dysarthria or a wet quality to the voice, which may indicate a laryngeal and neurologic condition, respectively. A neurologic examination should be performed to assess general evidence of neurologic dysfunction.

Testing and Referral

The relevant findings on history and physical examination will direct the appropriate testing or referrals for each patient with dysphagia (**Fig. 1**).

To determine the necessary steps in defining and treating each patient with dysphagia, it is important to decipher whether the complaints are consistent with supraesophageal symptoms. If the patient has signs of aspiration, especially with swallowing, or nasopharyngeal regurgitation, oropharyngeal dysphagia is suggested.

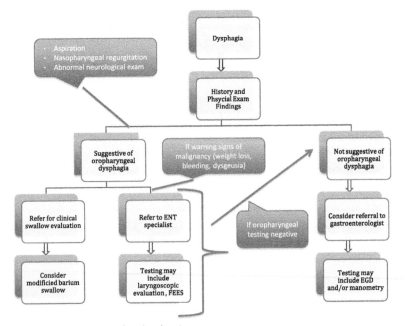

Fig. 1. Referrals and testing for dysphagia.

In this case, an appropriate initial test may be a clinical swallow evaluation, which typically is performed by a speech pathologist. During the examination, patients are given boluses of varying size and complexity.[14] Studies have found that such assessments can miss up to 50% of significant aspiration that is seen on videofluroroscopy.[15] Therefore, patients also generally undergo a modified barium swallow, which is a radiographic examination during which the patient is given foods of varying consistencies to assess dysphagia and aspiration.

Potential warning signs of malignancy, such as sudden weight loss, dysgeusia, or bleeding seen in a patient with oropharyngeal dysphagia, should lead to a referral to an ENT specialist. Besides a through head and neck evaluation, the ENT physician will also perform a laryngoscopic evaluation of the pharynx and larynx to look for tumors or other anatomic changes in the oropharynx, such as Zenker's diverticulum. Furthermore, the ENT physician may also perform a fiber optic endoscopic evaluation of swallowing (FEES), during which the patient is fed foods of varying consistencies, which are often colored for the purpose of visualization to assess swallowing function.[16] This evaluation is followed by endoscopic evaluation to check for food residue and entry of food particles into the larynx. If warning signs are present, computerized tomography may also be performed to rule out malignancy.

If the patient does not present with supraesophageal symptoms or if modified barium swallow/FEES study is negative, a barium video esophagram and gastroenterology referral should be considered. In some practices, a barium esophagram focuses primarily on the esophagus, although, in others, detailed attention is appropriately given to oropharyngeal swallowing. Appropriate esophageal radiography should include evaluation of not only the anatomy but also motility and function of the esophagus. In conjunction with fluoroscopic imaging, the patient swallows a barium suspension, which allows for visualization. It is often helpful to administer a solid bolus or barium tablet to assess for localized narrowing and temporal association of symptoms and holdup. Obstructions, such as esophageal strictures and tumors, can be seen, and even motility disorders such as achalasia can be suggested.[17] Because of its relatively low cost and simplicity, a barium esophagram is often recommended as the first-line test in a patient with likely esophageal dysphagia.[18]

As mentioned, referral to a gastroenterologist is appropriate if a patient has symptoms implying esophageal dysphagia. The specialist can perform an esophago-gastroduodenoscopy (EGD) or esophageal manometry, as indicated. An EGD is an endoscopic direct examination of the esophagus, stomach, and duodenum and can diagnose esophagitis, rings, webs, strictures, and tumors. If the patient's symptoms, such as long-term, chronic dysphagia, suggest esophageal dysmotility, esophageal manometry can be performed to help diagnose achalasia.[18] This procedure is performed by placing a thin catheter through the nose into the esophagus and assessing peristalsis in response to sips of water.

SPECIFIC DISORDERS

It is beyond the scope of this article to discuss every entity that causes dysphagia, but we discuss some of the most common disorders, especially those that disproportionately affect the elderly.

Oropharyngeal Dysphagia

Neuromuscular disorders

The most common causes of oropharyngeal dysphagia are of neurologic origin (**Box 2**).[19] Although an exact diagnosis can occasionally be made, this is not typically

---

Box 2
Disorders causing oropharyngeal dysphagia

Neuromuscular Causes

- Stroke
- Myasthenia gravis
- Parkinson's disease
- Amyotrophic lateral sclerosis (ALS)
- Multiple sclerosis (MS)
- Huntington's disease
- UES dysfunction
- Muscular dystrophy
- Other disorders of striated muscle

Structural Causes

- Head and neck tumors
- Zenker's diverticulum
- Cricopharyngeal bar/cricopharyngeal achalasia
- Osteophytes and other extrinsic causes

---

so. Furthermore, even if a neurologic disorder is diagnosed, often there is no specific treatment. However, certain disorders do lend themselves to a specific treatment; for example, anticholinesterase inhibitors are helpful in myasthenia gravis. Hence, if identified, it is important to treat the underlying neurologic disorder to improve dysphagia.[10]

Stroke is a common cause of dysphagia in the elderly. Importantly, each stroke patient should be clinically evaluated for signs of dysphagia and aspiration. Such swallowing dysfunction causes substantial morbidity and mortality, as it is estimated that approximately 50,000 stroke victims die each year in the United States from aspiration pneumonia related to dysphagia.[19] Studies show that more than 50% of all stroke patients will show clinical and fluoroscopic signs of dysphagia.[20] However, most stroke patients will regain healthy swallowing function within 1 or 2 weeks after infarction.[19]

Neurodegenerative diseases also play a large role in the increased frequency of dysphagia in the elderly population. Parkinson's disease, a disorder related to the degeneration of cells responsible for dopamine synthesis, causes widespread motor difficulties and tremor.[21] As symptoms of Parkinson's disease worsen, the risk of aspiration increases as a result of increased oropharyngeal transit time, among other factors.[22] Typically, the motor symptoms in Parkinson's disease are treated with the dopamine precursor L-DOPA, but the medication does not have the same efficacy in eliminating dysphagia. Other neuromuscular diseases that can cause dysphagia are listed in **Box 2**.

In most cases of neuromuscular-related oropharyngeal dysphagia, referral to a speech therapist is extremely helpful.[23] After appropriate clinical evaluation and examination, including either modified barium swallow or FEES study, the speech therapist will develop a treatment plan specific to the patient. Certain food consistencies can be eliminated from the diet, meal and bolus size can be adjusted, and swallowing techniques like the chin-tuck, head-turn, and supraglottic maneuvers can be used to avoid aspiration, enabling the patient to eat more comfortably and safely.[24,25] Dysphagia rehabilitation can also involve strengthening and coordinating muscles involved in swallowing using techniques such as the basic hard swallow, the Mendelsohn maneuver, and the Shaker head lift.[26] In the Mendelsohn maneuver, when a patient initiates a swallow, he holds the larynx at its highest point. This maneuver can increase muscle strength, swallow effort, and endurance. In the Shaker head lift, the patient is instructed to lie supine and lift the head up to look at the feet, holding this position for 1 minute. This exercise, in conjunction with sets of rapid head lifts, is performed over a 6-week period and has been found to significantly decrease aspiration. Of course, in some patients, no therapy can stop aspiration. In these unfortunate cases, artificial feeding, such as a gastrostomy tube, is considered as a last resort.

Structural disorders

Oropharyngeal structural disorders represent other causes of dysphagia in the elderly. These abnormalities, including Zenker's diverticulum, cricopharyngeal bar and achalasia, and tumors require specific treatment, but patients may also benefit from dysphagia rehabilitation guided by a speech pathologist.

Zenker's diverticula are increased in the elderly. They occur at Killian's triangle, which is located posteriorly in the pharynx between the inferior constrictor and cricopharyngeus muscles. These diverticula are typically diagnosed by esophagram. The precise cause of Zenker's diverticulum is still a subject of debate, but one prominent theory posits that it is caused by incomplete relaxation of the UES.[27] Indeed, the surgical treatment is primarily cricopharyngeal myotomy, currently typically performed through the oral route. Larger diverticula may also require diverticulopexy or, rarely, resection. Patients with mild symptoms or substantial comorbid conditions may benefit from dilation of the sphincter, foregoing surgery.[28] Sometimes, a radiologic cricopharyngeal bar, representing a poorly opening UES, may cause symptoms even in the absence of a Zenker's diverticulum. Such patients may also benefit from endoscopic dilation.

Head and neck tumors are a common structural cause of solid food dysphagia in the elderly. Patients with these tumors often have a notable history of smoking and alcohol use and are typically treated by an otolaryngologist, oncologist, and radiation oncologist. Dysphagia can lead to malnutrition and decreased quality of life in these patients, which both contribute to a poorer prognosis.[29] Dysphagia is often not relieved by surgical excision of the tumor, radiation therapy, or chemotherapy. Approximately 50% of patients still suffer from long-term oropharyngeal dysphagia after these treatments.[30] Swallow rehabilitation is important in these patients, because their dysphagia is often long lasting.

Esophageal Dysphagia

Structural disorders

Esophageal webs and rings are benign esophageal narrowings that may cause dysphagia (**Box 3**). An esophageal web is a mucosal and submucosal folding that causes obstruction and may rarely be associated with iron deficiency, as seen in Plummer-Vinson syndrome.[31] Esophageal rings are smooth mucosal constrictions that are seen on either esophagram or endoscopy. When located at the gastroesophageal junction, they are referred to as Schatzki rings, a very common cause of intermittent solid food dysphagia.[32] If multiple rings are seen, eosinophilic esophagitis should be considered. Vascular compression of the esophagus, including dysphagia lusoria and dysphagia aortica, also causes dysphagia.[33]

A peptic stricture is another benign esophageal narrowing that causes dysphagia and is common in the geriatric population. These strictures most often result from

---

Box 3
Disorders causing esophageal dysphagia

Structural Causes

- Esophageal webs
- Esophageal rings, including Schatzki rings
- Peptic and other strictures
- Esophageal malignancies
- Vascular compression and other extrinsic causes

Functional Causes

- Inflammatory disorders including erosive esophagitis
- Eosinophilic esophagitis (EoE)
- Achalasia
- DES
- Nutcracker esophagus
- Hypertensive LES
- Ineffective esophageal motility
- Scleroderma and other rheumatologic disorders

---

chronic inflammation from prolonged acid reflux. Heller myotomy for treatment of achalasia, prolonged nasogastric tube placement, and scleroderma increase the risk of peptic stricture formation. With a mild stricture, patients typically have difficulty only with solid foods. As the stricture progresses, patients begin to have difficulty with softer foods and even with liquids. Appropriate treatment involves controlling the patient's reflux and endoscopic esophageal dilation.[34]

Esophageal malignancies are more common in the elderly, and patients often present with rapidly progressive dysphagia. Typically, the prognosis is poor if the diagnosis of cancer is made after the manifestation of dysphagia, because the cancer has already progressed.[35] Malignancies leading to esophageal dysphagia include primary esophageal adenocarcinoma, squamous cell carcinoma, and adenocarcinoma of the gastroesophageal junction/cardia. Esophageal adenocarcinoma often occurs in patients with longstanding gastroesophageal reflux disease (GERD) via development of Barrett's metaplasia and dysplasia.[36,37] Esophageal squamous cell carcinoma typically occurs in patients with a significant smoking and alcohol history. These patients' treatments are typically coordinated by a gastroenterologist, surgeon, and medical and radiation oncologists.[38]

Functional disorders

Esophageal inflammation is a common cause of dysphagia. Inflammatory complications arising from GERD, including erosive esophagitis, are a common cause of dysphagia in this subgroup.[39] If the patient's dysphagia is reflux related, treating the reflux itself can often improve the symptoms. Eosinophilic esophagitis is an inflammatory cause of dysphagia that is becoming increasingly prevalent.[40] It is present in patients of all ages and can be responsible for dysphagia in an elderly patient.[41] Eosinophilic esophagitis often results in food impaction.[42] Other inflammatory causes of esophageal dysphagia include infection, caustic ingestion, radiation, and pill esophagitis.

Several esophageal motility disorders lead to dysphagia, with achalasia being the best-described condition. These motility disorders are best diagnosed by esophageal manometry but are often initially suggested by esophageal imaging studies. Achalasia is defined as incomplete LES relaxation combined with a lack of peristalsis.[43] Patients have difficulty swallowing both liquid and solid foods; they often have concurrent chest pain and weight loss. Achalasia is prevalent in about 1 in 10,000, but it is important to identify and treat appropriately. The 2 primary treatment modalities for achalasia are endoscopic pneumatic balloon dilation and myotomy.[44] However, in the elderly with comorbid conditions, it is often most appropriate to forego such risky procedures and perform only botulinum toxin injection or mild endoscopic dilation.

Many other motility disorders cause dysphagia.[45] Diffuse esophageal spasm (DES) is a disorder with intermingled normal peristalsis and simultaneous contractions. DES can result in chest pain and intermittent dysphagia; it may be primary or secondary to reflux. Nutcracker esophagus is characterized by high amplitude peristaltic contractions in the distal esophagus, and hypertensive LES is characterized by a high resting LES pressure. Both of these motility disorders also may present with chest pain and dysphagia. Ineffective esophageal motility disorder is a manometric diagnosis of low-amplitude peristaltic contractions and can also cause dysphagia; the etiology is typically reflux. Finally, scleroderma can cause aperistalsis or low-amplitude esophageal contractions as well as a hypotensive LES. Both solid and liquid food dysphagia are seen in these patients, and many scleroderma patients have strictures secondary to reflux.[46]

SUMMARY

Dysphagia, or difficulty with the normal swallowing process, is a common problem in the elderly. Patients with dysphagia can have predominantly oropharyngeal symptoms, esophageal symptoms, or a combination of both. A good clinical history and physical examination can suggest the need for further testing in each particular patient with dysphagia. The most common causes of oropharyngeal dysphagia are of neurologic origin, and clinical swallow examinations, in conjunction with an ENT specialist if warning signs imply malignancy, are important in the workup and treatment decisions for these patients. If a patient has likely esophageal dysphagia, a barium esophagram is often the initial appropriate test, but referral to a gastrointestinal specialist for opinion, endoscopy, or manometry is often required.

REFERENCES

1. Reynolds J, George B. Dysphagia. In: Pitchumoni CS, Dharmarajan TS, editors. Geriatric gastroenterology. New York: Springer; 2012. p. 293–300.
2. Ekberg O, Feinberg MJ. Altered swallowing function in elderly patients without dysphagia: radiologic findings in 56 cases. Am J Roentgenol 1991;156(6):1181–4.
3. Day JC. Population projections of the United States by age, sex, race, and Hispanic origin: 1995 to 2050, U.S. Bureau of the Census, Current Population Reports. Washington, DC: U.S. Government Printing Office; 1996. p. 25–1130. Available at: http://www.census.gov/prod/1/pop/p25-1130/p251130.pdf.
4. US Census Bureau. The older population in the United States: 2010 to 2050. Available at: http://www.census.gov/prod/2010pubs/p25-1138.pdf. Accessed August, 2013.
5. Carrión S, Verin E, Clavé P, et al. Complications of oropharyngeal dysphagia: malnutrition and aspiration pneumonia. In: Ekberg O, editor. Dysphagia. Berlin, New York: Springer; 2012. p. 575–99.

6. Norman K, Pichard C, Lochs H, et al. Prognostic impact of disease-related malnutrition. Clin Nutr 2008;27(1):5–15.

7. Persson MD, Brismar KE, Katzarski KS, et al. Nutritional status using mini nutritional assessment and subjective global assessment predict mortality in geriatric patients. J Am Geriatr Soc 2002;50(12):1996–2002.

8. Schindler JS, Kelly JH. Swallowing disorders in the elderly. Laryngoscope 2002; 112(4):589–602.

9. Furness JB. The enteric nervous system and neurogastroenterology. Nature reviews. Gastroenterol Hepatol 2012;9(5):286–94.

10. Sura L, Madhavan A, Carnaby G, et al. Dysphagia in the elderly: management and nutritional considerations. Clin Interv Aging 2012;7:287–98.

11. Cook IJ. Oropharyngeal dysphagia. Gastroenterol Clin North Am 2009;38(3):411–31.

12. Aviv JE, Martin JH, Jones ME, et al. Age-related changes in pharyngeal and supraglottic sensation. Ann Otol Rhinol Laryngol 1994;103(10):749–52.

13. Roy N, Stemple J, Merrill RM, et al. Dysphagia in the elderly: preliminary evidence of prevalence, risk factors, and socioemotional effects. Ann Otol Rhinol Laryngol 2007;116(11):858–65.

14. Marques CH, de Rosso AL, Andre C. Bedside assessment of swallowing in stroke: water tests are not enough. Top Stroke Rehabil 2008;15(4):378–83.

15. Splaingard ML, Hutchins B, Sulton LD, et al. Aspiration in rehabilitation patients: videofluoroscopy vs bedside clinical assessment. Arch Phys Med Rehabil 1988; 69(8):637–40.

16. Umay EK, Unlu E, Saylam GK, et al. Evaluation of dysphagia in early stroke patients by bedside, endoscopic, and electrophysiological methods. Dysphagia 2013;28(3):395–403.

17. Cho YK, Choi MG, Oh SN, et al. Comparison of bolus transit patterns identified by esophageal impedance to barium esophagram in patients with dysphagia. Dis Esophagus 2012;25(1):17–25.

18. Spieker MR. Evaluating dysphagia. Am Fam Physician 2000;61(12):3639–48.

19. Dray TG, Hillel AD, Miller RM. Dysphagia caused by neurologic deficits. Otolaryngol Clin North Am 1998;31(3):507–24.

20. Mann G, Hankey GJ, Cameron D. Swallowing function after stroke: prognosis and prognostic factors at 6 months. Stroke 1999;30(4):744–8.

21. Shulman JM, De Jager PL, Feany MB. Parkinson's disease: genetics and pathogenesis. Annu Rev Pathol 2011;6:193–222.

22. Nagaya M, Kachi T, Yamada T, et al. Videofluorographic study of swallowing in Parkinson's disease. Dysphagia 1998;13(2):95–100.

23. Rosenvinge SK, Starke ID. Improving care for patients with dysphagia. Age Ageing 2005;34(6):587–93.

24. Smith SK, Roddam H, Sheldrick H. Rehabilitation or compensation: time for a fresh perspective on speech and language therapy for dysphagia and Parkinson's disease? Int J Lang Commun Disord 2012;47(4):351–64.

25. Boden K, Hallgren A, Witt Hedstrom H. Effects of three different swallow maneuvers analyzed by videomanometry. Acta Radiol 2006;47(7):628–33.

26. Burkhead LM, Sapienza CM, Rosenbek JC. Strength-training exercise in dysphagia rehabilitation: principles, procedures, and directions for future research. Dysphagia 2007;22(3):251–65.

27. Watemberg S, Landau O, Avrahami R. Zenker's diverticulum: reappraisal. Am J Gastroenterol 1996;91(8):1494–8.

28. Veenker EA, Andersen PE, Cohen JI. Cricopharyngeal spasm and Zenker's diverticulum. Head Neck 2003;25(8):681–94.

29. Grobbelaar EJ, Owen S, Torrance AD, et al. Nutritional challenges in head and neck cancer. Clin Otolaryngol Allied Sci 2004;29(4):307–13.
30. Garcia-Peris P, Paron L, Velasco C, et al. Long-term prevalence of oropharyngeal dysphagia in head and neck cancer patients: impact on quality of life. Clin Nutr 2007;26(6):710–7.
31. Hoffman RM, Jaffe PE. Plummer-Vinson syndrome. A case report and literature review. Arch Intern Med 1995;155(18):2008–11.
32. Jalil S, Castell DO. Schatzki's ring: a benign cause of dysphagia in adults. J Clin Gastroenterol 2002;35(4):295–8.
33. Janssen M, Baggen MG, Veen HF, et al. Dysphagia lusoria: clinical aspects, manometric findings, diagnosis, and therapy. Am J Gastroenterol 2000;95(6): 1411–6.
34. Siersema PD, de Wijkerslooth LR. Dilation of refractory benign esophageal strictures. Gastrointest Endosc 2009;70(5):1000–12.
35. Villaflor VM, Allaix ME, Minsky B, et al. Multidisciplinary approach for patients with esophageal cancer. World J Gastroenterol 2012;18(46):6737–46.
36. Lieberman DA, Oehlke M, Helfand M. Risk factors for Barrett's esophagus in community-based practice. GORGE consortium. Gastroenterology Outcomes Research Group in Endoscopy. Am J Gastroenterol 1997;92(8):1293–7.
37. Pera M, Cameron AJ, Trastek VF, et al. Increasing incidence of adenocarcinoma of the esophagus and esophagogastric junction. Gastroenterology 1993;104(2): 510–3.
38. Sgourakis G, Gockel I, Lang H. Endoscopic and surgical resection of T1a/T1b esophageal neoplasms: a systematic review. World J Gastroenterol 2013;19(9): 1424–37.
39. Triadafilopoulos G. Nonobstructive dysphagia in reflux esophagitis. Am J Gastroenterol 1989;84(6):614–8.
40. Dellon ES, Gonsalves N, Hirano I, et al. ACG clinical guideline: evidenced based approach to the diagnosis and management of esophageal eosinophilia and eosinophilic esophagitis (EoE). Am J Gastroenterol 2013;108(5):679–92 [quiz: 693].
41. Prasad GA, Talley NJ, Romero Y, et al. Prevalence and predictive factors of eosinophilic esophagitis in patients presenting with dysphagia: a prospective study. Am J Gastroenterol 2007;102(12):2627–32.
42. Straumann A, Bussmann C, Zuber M, et al. Eosinophilic esophagitis: analysis of food impaction and perforation in 251 adolescent and adult patients. Clin Gastroenterol Hepatol 2008;6(5):598–600.
43. Michael FV, John EP, Marcelo FV. ACG clinical guideline: diagnosis and management of achalasia. Am J Gastroenterol 2013;108(8):1238–49.
44. Stavropoulos SN, Friedel D, Modayil R, et al. Endoscopic approaches to treatment of achalasia. Therap Adv Gastroenterol 2013;6(2):115–35.
45. Lacy BE, Weiser K. Esophageal motility disorders: medical therapy. J Clin Gastroenterol 2008;42(5):652–8.
46. Ntoumazios SK, Voulgari PV, Potsis K, et al. Esophageal involvement in scleroderma: gastroesophageal reflux, the common problem. Semin Arthritis Rheum 2006;36(3):173–81.

Microscopic Colitis

Darrell S. Pardi, MD, MS

KEYWORDS

- Microscopic colitis • Collagenous colitis • Lymphocytic colitis

KEY POINTS

- Microscopic colitis is a relatively common cause of chronic diarrhea, particularly in older adults.
- After a period of increasing incidence in the United States and Europe, it seems to be stabilizing.
- Colon biopsies are required for diagnosis and should be performed in any patient undergoing colonoscopy to evaluate chronic watery diarrhea.
- The 2 subtypes of microscopic colitis, collagenous and lymphocytic colitis, are similar histologically and clinically and seem to respond similarly to various medical therapies.
- Although there are few controlled trials of therapies for microscopic colitis, the treatment approach presented here often leads to satisfactory control of symptoms, although maintenance therapy is often required.

INTRODUCTION

Microscopic colitis is a relatively common cause of diarrhea, especially in the elderly. Overall, approximately 10% to 15% of patients investigated for chronic watery diarrhea are found to have this diagnosis, although this proportion is much higher in older patients. The diarrhea is often accompanied by other symptoms such as abdominal pain, and therefore, it is difficult to distinguish microscopic colitis from the more common irritable bowel syndrome (IBS) without colonic biopsies. The pathophysiology of microscopic colitis is not well established. Several treatment options are available, although few have been subjected to well-done clinical trials. This article reviews details of these issues.

CLINICAL FINDINGS

Microscopic colitis is characterized by chronic or intermittent watery diarrhea.[1] The severity of diarrhea can range from mild to severe with dehydration and electrolyte abnormalities. Other symptoms are often present, including abdominal pain, weight loss,

Disclosures: Consulting: Santarus.
Division of Gastroenterology and Hepatology, Inflammatory Bowel Disease Clinic, Mayo Clinic College of Medicine, 200 First Street SW, Rochester, MN 55905, USA
E-mail address: Pardi.darrell@mayo.edu

Clin Geriatr Med 30 (2014) 55–65
http://dx.doi.org/10.1016/j.cger.2013.10.005
0749-0690/14/$ – see front matter © 2014 Elsevier Inc. All rights reserved.

and arthralgias, each present in approximately 50% of patients. The weight loss is typically mild but can be significant in some cases. Quality of life is affected in proportion to the degree of diarrhea, abdominal pain, urgency, and incontinence.[2]

It is important to recognize that the symptoms of microscopic colitis are nonspecific. In fact, many patients with microscopic colitis meet the diagnostic criteria for IBS, such as the Manning or Rome criteria.[3] Therefore, these criteria are not specific, and histologic analysis of colon biopsies is required to distinguish microscopic colitis from the much more common IBS.

Microscopic colitis is an umbrella term that encompasses 2 main subtypes: collagenous colitis and lymphocytic colitis. These subtypes have very similar clinical and epidemiologic features, and the main distinction is histologic, as discussed below in the Diagnosis section. Given the significant clinical and histologic overlap between the 2 reports of patients transitioning from one type to the other over time or even having evidence for both types on biopsies from a single colonoscopy, and the similar response to treatments as discussed below in the Treatment section, it is not clear whether lymphocytic and collagenous colitis are 2 separate entities or part of a single disorder.[4] The current approach to these diagnoses is to consider them variants of the same condition.

The colonic mucosa generally appears endoscopically normal, although occasionally mild findings, such as edema or erythema, may be seen. Gross ulcerations suggest an alternate diagnosis, although these can be seen in patients with microscopic colitis who are taking nonsteroidal anti-inflammatory drugs (NSAIDs). Arthralgias are commonly present, and some patients also have increased erythrocyte sedimentation rates or positive results in tests for antinuclear antibodies or other markers of autoimmunity,[5] although these markers are insensitive and nonspecific for microscopic colitis.

Concomitant autoimmune conditions, such as diabetes mellitus, thyroid dysfunction, connective tissue disorders, and psoriasis, occur commonly in patients with microscopic colitis.[5,6] In particular, the association between microscopic colitis and celiac disease is clinically important. As many as 33% of patients with celiac disease have colonic histologic changes that are consistent with microscopic colitis.[7] In a large cohort study of patients with celiac disease, 4.3% were diagnosed with microscopic colitis, 72-fold greater than for patients without celiac disease.[8] Microscopic colitis is therefore more common among patients with celiac disease, and it should be considered in patients who have continued or recurrent diarrhea despite a strict gluten-free diet.[9]

On the other hand, the prevalence of celiac-like changes in the small bowel of patients with microscopic colitis ranges from 2% to 9% in the largest studies reporting this association.[5,6,10] However, in patients with microscopic colitis, celiac serologies are often negative, with anti-endomysial antibodies and anti-tissue transglutaminase antibodies being reported in 0% to 4%.[11,12] Therefore, serologies do not appear to be good diagnostic tools for celiac disease in patients with microscopic colitis. Finally, HLA types of patients with microscopic colitis were similar to those of patients with celiac disease in one study,[12] but not in others.

These data indicate that celiac disease is relatively uncommon in patients with microscopic colitis, and it is probably not necessary to evaluate these patients routinely for celiac disease. However, celiac disease should be considered in patients with features of malabsorption, such as significant weight loss, steatorrhea, and unexplained iron deficiency anemia, as well as those who do not respond to usual therapies, as discussed below in the Treatment section.

There have been a few reports of patients with microscopic colitis later developing inflammatory bowel disease (IBD) and of patients with IBD developing collagenous colitis. However, given the small number of cases, these reports could represent random chance associations. It also is important to recognize that histologic features of IBD, such as Paneth cells metaplasia and distortion of the crypt architecture, may occur in patients with microscopic colitis who otherwise have no evidence of IBD.[13]

The reported natural history of microscopic colitis varies considerably. The rate of symptomatic remission ranges from 59% to 93% in patients with lymphocytic colitis and 2% to 92% in those with collagenous colitis.[1] One study reported spontaneous remission in 15% of patients with collagenous colitis and treatment-induced remission in another 48%.[14] Only 22% required prolonged therapy. In contrast, clinical trials have reported that only 12% to 40% of patients respond to placebo after 6 to 8 weeks,[15–18] and an open-label study of steroid therapy reported that 90% of patients required maintenance therapy.[19]

EPIDEMIOLOGY

Microscopic colitis can develop in patients of any age, including children, but most commonly presents in older adults and the elderly. It is a relatively common finding among patients who undergo colonoscopy with biopsy for evaluation of chronic watery diarrhea, present in 10% to 15% of such patients.[10,20,21] In the elderly, this proportion is even higher.[10] Thus, microscopic colitis should be considered in all patients being evaluated for chronic diarrhea, especially in older patients.

Population-based studies in Europe and North America have reported the incidence of microscopic colitis to be between 1 and 12 per 100,000 person-years.[10,21–25] The reported incidence of collagenous colitis varies from 1.1 to 5.2 per 100,000 person-years and the incidence of lymphocytic colitis from 3.1 to 5.5 per 100,000 person-years.[10,21–25] Several studies reported the overall incidence of microscopic colitis and its subtypes to have increased substantially over time. For example, in a North American study, the incidence of microscopic colitis increased almost 20-fold, from 1.1 per 100,000 person-years to 19.6 per 100,000 person-years, from 1985 to 2001.[24] By the end of the study period, on December 31, 2001, the prevalence of microscopic colitis was 103.0 per 100,000 persons (39.3 for collagenous colitis and 63.7 for lymphocytic colitis).[24] Similarly, a European study reported that the incidence of microscopic colitis increased from 6.8 per 100,000 to 11.8 per 100,000 over a 6-year period.[10] The reasons for these increases in incidence are not clear, but increased awareness, with increasing use of colonoscopy with biopsies to evaluate patients with diarrhea, likely contributed. Indeed, the study from North America showed increasing use of colonoscopy in parallel with the increased incidence of microscopic colitis.

However, more recent data have shown a stabilization in the incidence rates. For example, follow-up data from Swedish and North American populations have shown a stabilization of incidence rates over the last 10 to 15 years.[26,27]

Although microscopic colitis can be diagnosed in patients of any age, it is more common among older individuals. The average age of patients at diagnosis ranges from 53 to 69 years.[6,10,21–23] A Canadian study found that patients older than 65 years were 5.6 times more likely to be diagnosed with microscopic colitis than younger persons.[25] On the other hand, pediatric cases have been reported, and in one study, 25% of patients were younger than 45 years of age.[6,28]

In most reports, microscopic colitis is more common in women than in men, with a female-to-male ratio in collagenous colitis ranging up to 9:1.[21,22,25] The gender ratio in lymphocytic colitis appears to be lower, and some studies reported no significant difference in rates between men and women.[21,24,25,29]

As opposed to other forms of chronic colitis, such as ulcerative colitis, there is no evidence that microscopic colitis is associated with an increased risk of colon cancer.[24,30] Cases of lung cancer have been reported in patients with collagenous colitis,[6,21,30,31] possibly reflecting an association with cigarette smoking, which may be more common in patients with collagenous colitis.[30–32] For example, one study reported that 25% of patients with collagenous colitis smoked cigarettes, compared with only 14% of patients with lymphocytic colitis.[31]

DIAGNOSIS

Grossly, the colon usually appears normal or has mild, nonspecific changes, such as erythema or edema. Colon ulcerations may occasionally be seen, typically reflecting NSAID use.[33] Fecal leukocytes can be present,[5] but are neither sensitive nor specific. Thus, the diagnosis of microscopic colitis relies on colonic histology.

The classic histologic finding in lymphocytic colitis is intraepithelial lymphocytosis (IEL),[31] defined arbitrarily as greater than 20 IEL per 100 epithelial cells. The IEL density is usually more prominent in the surface than the crypt epithelium. In addition, biopsies show a mixed infiltrate of acute and chronic inflammatory cells in the lamina propria. Collagenous colitis has similar inflammatory findings on colonic biopsies, although the IEL infiltrate tends to be less prominent. Therefore, the main distinguishing feature of collagenous colitis is a thickened subepithelial collagen layer. The collagen band thickness in patients with collagenous colitis varies substantially, from 7 to 100 μm, compared with a normal band of approximately 5 μm. In addition, biopsies often show surface epithelium damage including detachment of the epithelium in some cases. It is important to recognize that biopsies can contain neutrophils, with active cryptitis being reported in a third of patients,[13] although acute inflammation should not dominate the inflammatory infiltrate.

PATHOPHYSIOLOGY

The pathophysiology of microscopic colitis is not well understood. Existing mechanistic studies are typically small and often give conflicting results. Several hypotheses have been raised, with proposed mechanisms ranging from autoimmunity/immune dysregulation to a reaction to a luminal antigen such as various medications or infectious agents. It may be that the histologic finding that is currently labeled as "microscopic colitis" is the result of multiple different mechanisms with similar clinical and histologic features. Some of the proposed pathophysiologic mechanisms are discussed.

Genetic Predisposition

Several studies have investigated HLA associations and have found conflicting results. One study reported an HLA pattern similar to that seen in celiac sprue,[12] while another found no HLA association.[34] Abnormal HLA expression on colonocytes also has been described, suggesting that MHC-restricted immune activation could be involved.[35] However, given the conflicting results of these various studies, it is difficult to draw conclusions about the role of HLA haplotypes in microscopic colitis. Familial cases of microscopic colitis have been reported,[32] but the infrequency of this observation suggests that genetic predisposition is not a major factor in this disease.

Reaction to Luminal Antigen

This mechanism is suggested by studies of dietary factors, medications (see below in the Medication Side Effect section), or unspecified agents. For example, microscopic colitis is more common in patients with celiac sprue, and lymphocytic colitis-like changes can be induced in patients with sprue by a gluten enema.[36] Furthermore, symptoms and histologic changes of microscopic colitis may resolve with diversion of the fecal stream.[37] Finally, a lymphocytic colitis-like disorder in dogs resolves with a hypo-allergenic diet.[38] If microscopic colitis is due to an abnormal reaction to a luminal antigen, the immune reaction may have an autoimmune component, given the association with various autoimmune conditions and serologic markers.[11,34,39,40]

Abnormalities in Fluid Homeostasis

Several studies have reported abnormal fluid and electrolyte absorption or secretion in microscopic colitis,[41–43] although another reported normal absorption.[44] Abnormalities of the nitric oxide system[45] and prostaglandin levels[43] have been have been reported, suggesting possible mediators of abnormal secretion. The down-regulation of epithelial tight junction proteins may impair mucosal barrier function, contributing to passive fluid and electrolyte loss.[41]

Bile Acid Malabsorption

Several investigators have studied the role of bile acid malabsorption (BAM) in microscopic colitis, because patients with BAM (eg, after ileal resection) have diarrhea, and colonic infusion of bile acids in animals causes a colitis similar to lymphocytic colitis.[46] Villous atrophy, inflammation, and collagen deposition in the ileum have been reported in patients with microscopic colitis, suggesting a potential mechanism for BAM.[47] However, results of tests for BAM[42,44,47] have been conflicting, and many patients with normal results respond to a bile acid binder,[47] casting doubt on the validity of these tests or the importance of demonstrating BAM for directing therapy.

Infection

Several lines of evidence suggest the possibility of an infectious cause for microscopic colitis. Many patients with microscopic colitis have acute inflammation on biopsy and/or an acute onset of symptoms similar to a gastroenteritis,[4,44] and patients have been reported to respond to antibiotic therapy.[6] Furthermore, microscopic colitis has many features in common with "Brainerd diarrhea," a chronic diarrhea thought to be of infectious origin, which has mucosal lymphocytosis on colon biopsies.[48] Finally, a transgenic mouse model develops a lymphocytic colitis-like phenotype, but only if exposed to colonic bacteria.[49] However, no putative organism has been identified for microscopic colitis.

Medication Side Effect

An association between microscopic colitis and the use of NSAIDs has been reported in some studies but not in others, and some patients with microscopic colitis improve with discontinuation of NSAIDs.[14,50] Several other drugs also have been implicated as possible causes of microscopic colitis, including histamine-2 receptor blockers, carbamazepine, simvastatin, ticlopidine, flutamide, and others. One study assessed the strength of evidence that individual medications or classes of medications cause microscopic colitis and concluded that several drugs had strong evidence.[51] However, there are very few cases of positive drug rechallenge, and the number of cases for any specific drug is small, such that a chance association cannot be excluded. Furthermore, another study showed that some of the drug thought to cause microscopic colitis may simply worsen diarrhea, bringing subclinical cases to diagnosis, but do not actually cause the colitis.[52] Regardless, if a potential case of drug-induced microscopic colitis is identified, discontinuation of the offending medication may lead to symptom resolution.

Hormonal Influence

Microscopic colitis is more common in women, and there is a report of disease resolution during pregnancy,[6] raising the possibility of a hormonal influence, although this mechanism has not been well studied.

Abnormal Collagen Metabolism

Collagen typing studies have identified multiple potential abnormalities in patients with collagenous colitis.[53,54] Some studies suggest that the abnormal collagen layer is part of a reparative process in response to chronic inflammation, whereas others suggest a primary abnormality of collagen synthesis. Pericryptal fibroblasts regulate the production and deposition of basement membrane collagen.[55] In collagenous colitis, they appear to be activated with increased synthetic activity leading to excessive collagen production.[55] However, another study found no evidence for increased collagen synthesis as measured by messenger RNA levels[53] and others have not found elevated levels of fibroblast growth factor.

Transforming growth factor β may play a role in collagen deposition. This growth factor mediates collagen accumulation and, in one study, patients with collagenous colitis had increased expression of transforming growth factor β mRNA.[56] Vascular endothelial growth factor, another important mediator of fibrosis, appears to be upregulated in patients with collagenous colitis.[57] Furthermore, treatment with budesonide reduces vascular endothelial growth factor levels, at least in the lamina propria.[57]

It is likely that any abnormality of the fibroblast sheath is a secondary phenomenon, because it would not explain the inflammatory infiltrate. Furthermore, the severity of diarrhea in collagenous colitis is more strongly associated with the degree of inflammation and not with the thickness of the collagen band.[58]

In summary, various potential pathophysiologic mechanisms have been proposed in microscopic colitis. However, given the small number of patients studied in many of these reports, as well as the often contradictory findings, it is difficult to draw firm conclusions regarding the underlying pathophysiology of lymphocytic or collagenous colitis.

TREATMENT
Pharmacologic Treatment Options

The first step in managing patients with microscopic colitis is to search for exacerbating factors, including a careful dietary history searching for foods that might contribute to diarrhea, such as dairy products in a patient with lactose intolerance or excessive consumption of diet products that contain artificial sweeteners that can lead to diarrhea. It is also important to review the patient's medication list, including over-the-counter products and health food supplements, to search for drugs or other substances that might cause microscopic colitis or exacerbate diarrhea. In some patients, identification and elimination of such a factor may lead to improvement or even resolution of the diarrhea. However, most patients with microscopic colitis will require treatment.

Nonspecific antidiarrheal medications such as loperamide or diphenoxylate can be effective in patients with microscopic colitis[5,6,10] and are often used empirically in patients with mild diarrhea. If these medications are unsuccessful, or for patients with moderate symptoms, bismuth subsalicylate at a dose of 3 tablets (262 mg each) 3 times per day can be successful,[5,59] although one study found that most patients treated with this medication only experience partial response.[5] However, some patients who respond to this therapy achieve a long-lasting remission without maintenance therapy.[59]

For patients with diarrhea that does not respond to bismuth or those with severe symptoms, corticosteroids are typically used. In the largest, uncontrolled observational series, steroids have been the most effective therapies reported. Budesonide is the best-studied treatment for microscopic colitis, with 3 randomized, placebo-controlled induction studies in collagenous colitis[15–17] and 2 in lymphocytic colitis.[18,60] In all of these studies, budesonide was superior to placebo for inducing response, with response rates typically in the 80% to 90% range. Budesonide has fewer side effects than prednisone, and in one uncontrolled study it seemed to be more effective.[19] Therefore, unless cost is a significant concern, budesonide is generally used when corticosteroid therapy is necessary.

Despite the demonstrated efficacy of budesonide for induction, relapse is common (~70%) when it is discontinued.[10,19,61] Therefore, many patients become steroid dependent, and thus, before starting a patient on budesonide, the diagnosis should be reviewed and alternative diagnoses, such as concomitant celiac sprue, should be excluded if not done so already.

Immune suppressing medications such as azathioprine, 6-mercaptopurine, or methotrexate can be helpful in steroid-dependent or steroid-refractory patients.[5,62,63] However, to avoid the risks of immunosuppression, particularly in older patients, many clinicians are using long-term, low-dose budesonide (3–6 mg/d) for patients with steroid-dependent colitis.[64] This practice has been assessed in 2 randomized, placebo-controlled maintenance trials, which demonstrated that budesonide, 6 mg/d, was superior to placebo for maintaining response, at least through 6 months.[65,66] However, even after that duration of treatment, relapse was still high after budesonide was discontinued.

Therefore, if diarrhea recurs soon after completion of a successful course of budesonide (typically 9 mg/d given for 6–8 weeks), it is given again, often at a dose of 6 mg per day. Once remission is re-established, the dose is reduced to 3 mg per day, if possible and then to 3 mg every other day. After 6 to 12 months of therapy, another attempt is made to discontinue budesonide. If relapse occurs again, budesonide is restarted at the lowest effective dose.

Patients treated with long-term budesonide should be monitored for steroid-related side effects, such as hypertension, hyperglycemia, and metabolic bone disease, among others.[64] These patients should avoid consuming grapefruits and grapefruit juice, and any other cytochrome P450 inhibitors, which interfere with budesonide metabolism and predispose to side effects.

It is unusual for a patient not to respond to budesonide,[19] and in these patients, alternate or concomitant diagnoses and noncompliance should be considered. Treatment with an aminosalicylate is often considered as a treatment for these patients, or perhaps even before budesonide is used. However, several large uncontrolled series[5,6,10] have reported that only a minority of patients responds to aminosalicylates, and a recent placebo-controlled study in patients with collagenous colitis was negative.[67]

For patients that do have steroid-resistant microscopic colitis, treatment options include a bile acid binding agent or an immunomodulator, although there are relatively little data on these treatments. Cholestyramine can be effective,[5,6,10] although many patients do not tolerate it because of its texture. Bile-acid binders in tablet form, such as colesevalam or colestipol, might be better tolerated. There have been a few reports of the use of azathioprine,[62] methotrexate,[63] or anti-tumor necrosis factor therapies such as adalimumab and infliximab[68,69] in patients with steroid-refractory microscopic colitis.

Surgical Treatment Options

Patients rarely require surgery for medically refractory microscopic colitis. Reported operations include an ileostomy, with or without a colectomy,[5,37] or ileal pouch anal anastomosis.[70]

SUMMARY

Microscopic colitis is a relatively common cause of chronic diarrhea, particularly in older adults. After a period of increasing incidence in the United States and Europe, it seems to be stabilizing. Colon biopsies are required for diagnosis and should be performed in any patient undergoing colonoscopy to evaluate chronic watery diarrhea. The 2 subtypes of microscopic colitis, collagenous and lymphocytic colitis, are similar histologically and clinically, and seem to respond similarly to various medical therapies. Although there are few controlled trials of therapies for microscopic colitis, the treatment approach presented here often leads to satisfactory control of symptoms, although maintenance therapy is often required.

REFERENCES

1. Pardi DS, Kelly C. Microscopic colitis. Gastroenterology 2011;140:1155–65.
2. Madisch A, Heymer P, Voss C, et al. Oral budesonide therapy improves quality of life in patients with collagenous colitis. Int J Colorectal Dis 2005;20:312–6.
3. Limsui D, Pardi DS, Camilleri M, et al. Symptomatic overlap between irritable bowel syndrome and microscopic colitis. Inflamm Bowel Dis 2007;13:175–81.
4. Jessurun J, Yardley JH, Lee EL, et al. Microscopic and collagenous colitis: different names for the same condition? Gastroenterology 1986;91(6):1583–4.
5. Pardi DS, Ramnath VR, Loftus EV Jr, et al. Lymphocytic colitis: clinical features, treatment, and outcomes. Am J Gastroenterol 2002;97(11):2829–33.
6. Bohr J, Tysk C, Eriksson S, et al. Collagenous colitis: a retrospective study of clinical presentation and treatment in 163 patients. Gut 1996;39(6):846–51.
7. Wolber R, Owen D, Freeman H. Colonic lymphocytosis in patients with celiac sprue. Hum Pathol 1990;21:1092–6.
8. Green PH, Yang J, Cheng J, et al. An association between microscopic colitis and celiac disease. Clin Gastroenterol Hepatol 2009;7:1210–6.
9. Fine KD, Meyer RL, Lee EL. The prevalence and cause of chronic diarrhea in patients with celiac sprue treated with a gluten-free diet. Gastroenterology 1997;112:1830–8.
10. Olesen M, Eriksson S, Bohr J, et al. Microscopic colitis: a common diarrhoeal disease. An epidemiological study in Orebro, Sweden, 1993-1998. Gut 2004; 53(3):346–50.
11. Bohr J, Tysk C, Yang P, et al. Autoantibodies and immunoglobulins in collagenous colitis. Gut 1996;39(1):73–6.
12. Fine KD, Do K, Schulte K, et al. High prevalence of celiac sprue-like HLA-DQ genes and enteropathy in patients with the microscopic colitis syndrome. Am J Gastroenterol 2000;95:1974–82.
13. Ayata G, Ithamukkala S, Sapp H, et al. Prevalence and significance of inflammatory bowel disease-like morphological features in collagenous and lymphocytic colitis. Am J Surg Pathol 2002;26:1414–23.

14. Goff JS, Barnett JL, Pelke T, et al. Collagenous colitis: histopathology and clinical course. Am J Gastroenterol 1997;92:57–60.
15. Bonderup OK, Hansen JB, Birket-Smith L, et al. Budesonide treatment of collagenous colitis: a randomized, double-blind, placebo controlled trial with morphometric analysis. Gut 2003;52:248–51.
16. Baert F, Schmit A, D'Haens G, et al. Budesonide in collagenous colitis: a double-blind placebo-controlled trial with histologic follow-up. Gastroenterology 2002; 122:20–5.
17. Miehlke S, Heymer P, Bethke B, et al. Budesonide treatment for collagenous colitis: a randomized, double-blind, placebo-controlled, multicenter trial. Gastroenterology 2002;123:978–84.
18. Miehlke S, Madish A, Karimi D, et al. A randomized double-blind, placebo-controlled study showing that budesonide is effective in treating lymphocytic colitis. Gastroenterology 2009;136:2092–100.
19. Gentile N, Abdalla A, Khanna S, et al. Outcomes of patients with microscopic colitis treated with corticosteroids: a population-based study. Am J Gastroenterol 2013;108:256–9.
20. Fine KD, Seidel RH, Do K. The prevalence, anatomic distribution, and diagnosis of colonic causes of chronic diarrhea. Gastrointest Endosc 2000;51(3): 318–26.
21. Fernandez-Banares F, Salas A, Forne M, et al. Incidence of collagenous and lymphocytic colitis: a 5-year population-based study. Am J Gastroenterol 1999;94(2):418–23.
22. Bohr J, Tysk C, Eriksson S, et al. Collagenous colitis in Orebro, Sweden, an epidemiological study 1984-1993. Gut 1995;37(3):394–7.
23. Agnarsdottir M, Gunnlaugsson O, Orvar KB, et al. Collagenous and lymphocytic colitis in Iceland. Dig Dis Sci 2002;47(5):1122–8.
24. Pardi DS, Loftus EV Jr, Smyrk TC, et al. The epidemiology of microscopic colitis: a population based study in Olmsted County, Minnesota. Gut 2007; 56(4):504–8.
25. Williams JJ, Kaplan GG, Makhija S, et al. Microscopic colitis-defining incidence rates and risk factors: a population-based study. Clin Gastroenterol Hepatol 2008;6(1):35–40.
26. Gentile NM, Khanna S, Loftus EV Jr, et al. The epidemiology of microscopic colitis in Olmsted County from 2002 to 2010: a population-based study. Clin Gastroenterol Hepatol 2013. [Epub ahead of print]. http://dx.doi.org/10.1016/j.cgh.2013.09.066.
27. Wickbom A, Bohr J, Eriksson S, et al. Stable incidence of collagenous colitis and lymphocytic colitis in Örebro, Sweden, 1999–2008: a continuous epidemiologic study. Inflamm Bowel Dis 2013;19:2387–93.
28. Gremse DA, Boudreaux CW, Manci EA. Collagenous colitis in children. Gastroenterology 1993;104(3):906–9.
29. Olesen M, Eriksson S, Bohr J, et al. Lymphocytic colitis: a retrospective clinical study of 199 Swedish patients. Gut 2004;53(4):536–41.
30. Chan JL, Tersmette AC, Offerhaus GJ, et al. Cancer risk in collagenous colitis. Inflamm Bowel Dis 1999;5(1):40–3.
31. Baert F, Wouters K, D'Haens G, et al. Lymphocytic colitis: a distinct clinical entity? A clinicopathological confrontation of lymphocytic and collagenous colitis. Gut 1999;45(3):375–81.
32. Jarnerot G, Hertervig E, Granno C, et al. Familial occurrence of microscopic colitis: a report on five families. Scand J Gastroenterol 2001;36(9):959–62.

33. Kakar S, Pardi DS, Burgart LJ. Colonic ulcers accompanying collagenous colitis: implication of NSAIDs. Am J Gastroenterol 2003;98:1834–7.
34. Sylwestrowicz T, Kelly JK, Hwang WS, et al. Collagenous colitis and microscopic colitis: the watery diarrhea-colitis syndrome. Am J Gastroenterol 1989;84:763–8.
35. Beaugerie L, Luboinski J, Brousse N, et al. Drug induced lymphocytic colitis. Gut 1994;35:426–8.
36. Dobbins W, Rubin C. Studies of the rectal mucosa and celiac sprue. Gastroenterology 1964;47:471–9.
37. Jarnerot G, Tysk C, Bohr J, et al. Collagenous colitis and fecal stream diversion. Gastroenterology 1995;109:449–55.
38. Nelson RW, Stookey LJ, Kazacos E. Nutritional management of idiopathic chronic colitis in the dog. J Vet Intern Med 1988;2:133–7.
39. Giardiello FM, Lazenby AJ, Bayless TM, et al. Lymphocytic (microscopic) colitis. Clinicopathologic study of 18 patients and comparison to collagenous colitis. Dig Dis Sci 1989;34(11):1730–8.
40. Freeman HJ. Perinuclear antineutrophil cytoplasmic antibodies in collagenous or lymphocytic colitis with or without celiac disease. Can J Gastroenterol 1997;11:417–20.
41. Burgel N, Bojarski C, Mankertz J, et al. Mechanisms of diarrhea in collagenous colitis. Gastroenterology 2002;123(2):433–43.
42. Giardiello FM, Bayless TM, Jessurun J, et al. Collagenous colitis: physiologic and histopathologic studies in seven patients. Ann Intern Med 1987;106:46–9.
43. Rask-Madsen J, Grove O, Hansen MG, et al. Colonic transport of water and electrolytes in a patient with secretory diarrhea due to collagenous colitis. Dig Dis Sci 1983;28:1141–6.
44. Kingham JG, Levison DA, Ball JA, et al. Microscopic colitis—a cause of chronic watery diarrhea. Br Med J 1992;285:1601–4.
45. Lundberg JO, Herulf M, Olesen M, et al. Increased nitric oxide production in collagenous and lymphocytic colitis. Eur J Clin Invest 1997;27:869–71.
46. Chadwick VS, Gaginella TS, Carlson GL, et al. Effect of molecular structure on bile acid induced alterations in absorptive function, permeability and morphology in the perfused rabbit colon. J Lab Clin Med 1979;94:661–74.
47. Einarsson K, Eusufzai S, Johansson U, et al. Villous atrophy of distal ileum and lymphocytic colitis in a woman with bile acid malabsorption. Eur J Gastroenterol Hepatol 1992;4:585–90.
48. Osterholm MT, MacDonald KL, White KE, et al. An outbreak of a newly recognized chronic diarrhea syndrome associated with raw milk consumption. JAMA 1986;256:484–90.
49. Rath HC, Herfarth HH, Ikeda JS, et al. Normal luminal bacteria, especially Bacteroides species, mediate chronic colitis, gastritis, and arthritis in HLA B27/human beta 2 microglobulin transgenic rats. J Clin Invest 1996;98:945–53.
50. Riddell RH, Tanaka M, Mazzoleni G. Non-steroidal anti-inflammatory drugs as a possible cause of collagenous colitis: a case-control study. Gut 1992;33:683–6.
51. Beaugerie L, Pardi DS. Review article: drug-induced microscopic colitis—proposal for a scoring system and review of the literature. Aliment Pharmacol Ther 2005;22(4):277–84.
52. Fernandez Banarez F, Esteve M, Espinos JC, et al. Drug consumption and the risk of microscopic colitis. Am J Gastroenterol 2007;102:324–30.
53. Aigner T, Neureiter D, Muller S, et al. Extracellular matrix composition and gene expression in collagenous colitis. Gastroenterology 1997;113:136–43.

54. Gunther U, Schuppan D, Bauer M, et al. Fibrogenesis and fibrolysis in collagenous colitis. Am J Pathol 1999;155:493–503.
55. Hwang WS, Kelly JK. Collagenous colitis: a disease of pericryptal fibroblast sheath? J Pathol 1986;149:33–40.
56. Stahle-Backdahl M, Maim J, Veress B, et al. Increased presence of eosinophilic granulocytes expressing transforming growth factor-beta1 in collagenous colitis. Scand J Gastroenterol 2000;35(7):742–6.
57. Griga T, Tromm A, Schmiegel W, et al. Collagenous colitis: implications for the role of vascular endothelial growth factor in repair mechanisms. Eur J Gastroenterol Hepatol 2004;16(4):397–402.
58. Lee E, Schiller LR, Vendrell D, et al. Subepithelial collagen table thickness in colon specimens from patients with microscopic colitis and collagenous colitis. Gastroenterology 1992;103:1790–6.
59. Fine KD, Lee EL. Efficacy of open-label bismuth subsalicylate for the treatment of microscopic colitis. Gastroenterology 1998;114(1):29–36.
60. Pardi DS, Loftus EV, Tremaine WJ, et al. A randomized, double-blind, placebo-controlled trial of budesonide for the treatment of active lymphocytic colitis. Gastroenterology 2009;136:A519.
61. Miehlke S, Madisch A, Voss C, et al. Long-term follow-up of collagenous colitis after induction of clinical remission with budesonide. Aliment Pharmacol Ther 2005;22:1115–9.
62. Pardi DS, Loftus EV, Tremaine WJ, et al. Treatment of refractory microscopic colitis with azathioprine and 6-mercaptopurine. Gastroenterology 2001;120:1483–4.
63. Riddell J, Hillman L, Chiragakis L, et al. Collagenous colitis: oral low-dose methotrexate for patients with difficult symptoms: long-term outcomes. J Gastroenterol Hepatol 2007;22:1589–93.
64. Pardi DS. After budesonide, what next for collagenous colitis? Gut 2009;58:3–4.
65. Bonderup OK, Hansen JB, Teglbjoerg PS, et al. Long-term budesonide treatment of collagenous colitis: a randomised, double-blind, placebo-controlled trial. Gut 2009;58:68–72.
66. Miehlke S, Madish A, Bethke B, et al. Oral budesonide for maintenance treatment of collagenous colitis: a randomized, double-blind, placebo controlled trial. Gastroenterology 2008;135:1510–6.
67. Miehlke S, Madisch A, Kupcinskas L, et al. Double-blind, double-dummy, randomized, placebo-controlled, multicenter trial of Budesonide and mesalamine in collagenous colitis. Gastroenterology 2012;142(Suppl 1):S211.
68. Munch A, Ignatova S, Strom M. Adalimumab in budesonide and methotrexate refractory collagenous colitis. Scand J Gastroenterol 2012;47:59–63.
69. Esteve M, Mahadavan U, Sainz E, et al. Efficacy of anti-TNF therapies in refractory severe microscopic colitis. J Crohns Colitis 2011;5:612–8.
70. Varghese L, Galandiuk S, Tremaine WJ, et al. Lymphocytic colitis treated with proctocolectomy and ileal J-pouch anal anastomosis. Dis Colon Rectum 2002;45:123–6.

Medical Management of Inflammatory Bowel Disease in the Elderly: Balancing Safety and Efficacy

Christina Y. Ha, MD

KEYWORDS

- Inflammatory bowel disease • Infection • Polypharmacy • Adverse events
- Coordinated care

KEY POINTS

- Older patients are at an increased risk for adverse events with therapy because of the increased comorbidity, polypharmacy, and age-related physiologic changes affecting functional reserve and drug metabolism.
- Older patients with inflammatory bowel disease (IBD) are less able to tolerate the increased disease burden, with frequent hospitalizations because of gastrointestinal bleeding, malnutrition, electrolyte disturbances, and infection.
- Chronic steroids use is prevalent among older patients with IBD with lower rates of steroid-sparing regimens, such as thiopurines, or biologics, which may contribute to increased infection.
- Although biologics and immunomodulators may be associated with increased adverse event rates among the older patients with IBD, appropriate prescribing of these steroid-sparing agents earlier during the disease course may improve disease-related outcomes.
- Earlier recognition of disease flares and adverse events to therapy with heightened monitoring and coordinated care may lead to better outcomes.

INTRODUCTION

Approximately 10% of patients with inflammatory bowel disease (IBD) are older than 60 years.[1] The medical management of the older patient with IBD is more complex than younger patients because of the age-related pharmacokinetic changes in drug metabolism, preexisting comorbidity, polypharmacy, and potential medication interactions or contraindications. Aging is associated with numerous physiologic changes relating to organ system function and physical reserve, which affect drug metabolism and clearance. Changes in body fat percentage, serum protein, lean body mass, and total body water may alter plasma concentrations of lipophilic or hydrophilic

Division of Digestive Diseases, Center for Inflammatory Bowel Diseases, The David Geffen School of Medicine at UCLA, 200 Medical Plaza, Suite 365C, Los Angeles CA 90095, USA
E-mail address: cha@mednet.ucla.edu

Clin Geriatr Med 30 (2014) 67–78
http://dx.doi.org/10.1016/j.cger.2013.10.007
0749-0690/14/$ – see front matter © 2014 Elsevier Inc. All rights reserved.
geriatric.theclinics.com

medications, particularly with weight-based treatment regimens. Medication bioavailability and metabolism may be further impaired with aging because of decreased hepatic mass and decreased hepatic and renal blood flow, as well as glomerular filtration rate.[2] Therefore, conventional medication dosing and schedules may require adjustment when given to the older person.

Comorbidity also increases with age, because an estimated 20% of Medicare patients have 5 or more chronic conditions.[3] Alongside increasing comorbidity is a greater likelihood of polypharmacy, defined as the multiple use of medications by patients. Older Americans take more routine medications, including prescription medications, over-the-counter medications, supplements, and herbal therapies, than any other age group, making them more susceptible to medication-related adverse events (AEs) and drug interactions.[4] Greater than 50% of older patients take 5 or more medications on a regular basis, which increases the risk for drug-drug interactions and AEs.[5,6] Significant polypharmacy may affect medication adherence and lead to prescribing cascades. Prescribing cascades occur when an AE to therapy is considered as either a new symptom or an exacerbation of a preexisting condition leading to adjustments in dosages of the offending medication or the addition of another new medication to treat the symptom. This cycle may result in greater polypharmacy, AEs, and unnecessary or inappropriate medication prescribing.[7]

For the older patient with IBD, management often relies on the use of immunosuppressive agents or complex combinations of therapies in order to achieve disease control. The addition of immunosuppressive therapy to treat IBD in the older patient, considering the age-related variables and comorbidity, may affect therapeutic outcomes, including medication-related AEs, such as infection, malignancy, and mortality. Therefore, careful consideration of the risks, benefits, and alternatives of immunosuppression is necessary before medication prescribing with careful monitoring after initiation. In this review, the goals of medical therapy for older patients with IBD, prescribing patterns for geriatric patients with IBD, and methods to prevent the potential pitfalls of conventional IBD treatments in this more susceptible patient group are discussed.

Goals of Medical Therapy for Older Patients with IBD

The goals of therapy for IBD are similar across age groups: obtaining disease remission, the absence of clinical symptoms, ideally with healing of the affected mucosa, and maintaining symptom-free remission, with minimal AEs and decreased long-term disease-related complications. With sustained control of disease activity, there is the potential to modify the natural history of IBD by decreasing exposure to steroids, eliminating disability, and maintaining functional independence and avoiding hospitalizations and surgery.[8] These aspects of disease control are especially important for the older patient with IBD, who may be less able to recover from prolonged periods of disease activity.

IBD medication selection is typically dependent on disease severity, with more aggressive disease mandating the use of immunosuppressive medications such as corticosteroids, immunomodulators, or biologics. Based on clinical trial data, there has been a shift toward more of a top-down strategy, with earlier initiation of biological agents, such as the anti–tumor necrosis factor (anti-TNF) agents, either alone or in combination with thiopurines, to induce and maintain remission, because these therapies lead to higher rates of sustained remission, mucosal healing, and decreased disease-associated morbidity.[9–11] However, combinations of immunosuppression may also be associated with increased risk of infection and other medication-related AEs, particularly steroid-related combination therapy.[12,13]

Although therapeutic efficacy of the currently available IBD medications has been shown across multiple trials of these IBD agents, these findings may not be directly translated to the older patients with IBD, because the study populations were more representative of younger patients with IBD.

In addition to disease-specific symptoms, other age-specific variables need to be factored into the algorithms of IBD medical decision making for the older patient, particularly with respect to immunosuppression. Comorbid conditions such as smoking history, cardiopulmonary disease, diabetes, and cancer history are more prevalent among older persons, which may affect the natural history of their IBD and limit treatment options, because of known or potential contraindications and increased AE risk.[14,15] Numerous studies have suggested older age as an independent variable for increased risk of serious and opportunistic infections among patients with IBD.[12,13,16] Older patients may be inherently more susceptible to gastrointestinal infection, because of age-associated changes in the gastrointestinal flora and immune senescence.[17–19] *Clostridium difficile* infection, as an example, is associated with significant morbidity and mortality among older patients with IBD, with higher colectomy rates, longer hospital stays, and higher in-hospital mortality, particularly among those patients with higher comorbidity scores.[20] Pneumonia, sepsis, *Clostridium difficile* infection, and urinary tract infections are among the most common infection-related hospitalizations among patients with IBD, with older age and comorbidity being associated with increased risk.[21]

Although the older patient with IBD may be more susceptible to AEs of therapy than the younger person, older patients are also less able to tolerate severe or prolonged periods of disease activity. The loss of physical reserve associated with aging, changes in functional status, and increased susceptibility to falls may affect their disease course, as well as decreased sphincter function as a result of difficulties managing increased bowel frequency, nocturnal bowel movements, and increased incontinence.[22] Earlier control of disease activity with appropriate medications for the level of disease activity may optimize clinical status more rapidly, thus improving quality of life and decreasing hospitalization. However, when managing older patients with IBD, lower thresholds are needed to investigate changes in symptoms, such as increased diarrhea, fevers, or flulike symptoms, because they may represent early signs of infection-related complications of therapy. Appropriate vaccinations with the pneumococcal and influenza vaccine may decrease risk of serious infection, because the more common infectious AEs to therapy are vaccine preventable. Minimizing or avoiding prolonged antibiotic use; proper hand and stool hygiene; and prompt removal of indwelling catheters may also decrease infection potential among this more susceptible age group.

5-Aminosalicylate Treatment in the Elderly

The 5-aminosalicylate (5-ASA) medications are the mainstay of treatment of mild to moderate ulcerative colitis (UC) and, although there is little evidence to support their use in Crohn disease (CD), many older patients are maintained on 5-ASA therapy for their Crohn colitis.[23,24] Although these medications are generally considered safe and well tolerated across all age groups, certain considerations are important to remember when prescribing this class of medications for the older person, such as the daily pill burden, pill size, and dosing frequency. Because once-daily 5-ASA dosing has similar efficacy to the conventional split-dosing regimens, a simplified dosing schedule with lower total pill volumes may improve medication adherence and decrease risk of flaring.[25,26] In addition, 5-ASA–associated hypersensitivity may occur, with estimates of 3% to 10% of patients affected by this drug-related condition.

Symptoms of 5-ASA hypersensitivity may mimic colitis flares and resolve with discontinuation of the medication.[27] Topical therapies, including mesalamine enemas or suppositories, have been well-established adjuncts to oral 5-ASA agents for left-sided and extensive colitis as well as primary therapies for ulcerative proctitis.[28–30] However, anal resting tone decreases with age, and fecal incontinence is more prevalent among older persons.[31,32] Therefore, older persons may not be able to retain enemas as readily as younger patients, particularly during active disease.

Nephrotoxicity associated with 5-ASA is rare, occurring at a rate of 0.26% per patient year and manifesting as an idiosyncratic interstitial nephritis independent of 5-ASA dosing or duration of therapy.[33,34] Routine monitoring of renal function for all patients on 5-ASAs is recommended, although there is no established consensus as to the optimal surveillance schedule. Because glomerular filtration rate declines with age and many elderly persons either may have preexisting conditions that increase risk for renal insufficiency (eg, diabetes or hypertension) or may be taking potentially nephrotoxic medications, heightened monitoring may be warranted, particularly in the setting of chronic renal disease.

Corticosteroid Treatment in the Elderly

Corticosteroids are often used for induction of remission in the setting of 5-ASA refractory disease or moderate to severe disease activity. However, their role as a maintenance therapy has not been established, and chronic steroid use is linked to a multitude of potential AEs, particularly among older patients.[23,24] Steroid use has been associated with an increased risk of serious and opportunistic infections, worsened hypertension, diabetes, glaucoma and cataract formation, and mortality.[12,35,36] Older patients with IBD are already more susceptible to vitamin D deficiency, osteoporosis, and avascular necrosis. Prolonged steroid use only increases the fracture risk.[37,38] Because the older patient is particularly susceptible to these steroid-associated complications, it is of paramount importance for the practitioner to have a steroid-sparing exit strategy to decrease risk of these AEs and to avoid repeated courses or chronic use of steroids to treat the underlying IBD. Annual ophthalmologic examinations, adequate calcium plus vitamin D supplementation, and appropriate bone densitometry testing are recommended for patients with IBD exposed to chronic steroids.[39]

Immunomodulator Treatment in the Elderly

The thiopurines 6-mercaptopurine and azathioprine are commonly used as steroid-sparing maintenance medications for the treatment of IBD, and their longer-term efficacy has been established across clinical trials through the years.[40,41] However, therapeutic drug monitoring while on thiopurines is essential for the older patient with IBD, with routine checks for leukopenia and increases of liver enzyme levels. Before prescribing thiopurines to the older patient with IBD, a review of an updated medication list is necessary, because thiopurines may interact with several other classes of medications commonly prescribed by other members of their medical team, such as angiotensin-converting enzyme inhibitors and allopurinol, which result in increased myelotoxcity.[42] Mesalamines can also increase levels of therapeutic thiopurine metabolites because of inhibition of thiopurine methyltransferase enzyme activity by the 5-ASA, which may also increase risk for leukopenia.[43]

Prolonged thiopurine use has been associated with an increased risk of non-Hodgkin lymphoma.[44,45] According to data from the CESAME cohort study, the incidence rate of lymphoproliferative disorders among thiopurine users was approximately 9 cases per 10,000 patient years.[45] However, most (78%) patients diagnosed with lymphoma during the study period were older than 50 years. The patient subgroups who were at the greatest risk of lymphoma were the patients older than 65 years who were either currently taking thiopurines or were previously exposed to thiopurines.[45] Although this increased risk of lymphoma associated with thiopurines is not an absolute contraindication for its use among older patients with IBD, it should be considered when discussing potential steroid-sparing strategies. Thiopurines are also associated with an increased risk of nonmelanoma skin cancers, with the greatest risk again noted among older patients currently taking or previously exposed to immunomodulators.[46,47] Therefore, counseling regarding sun protection and routine dermatologic examinations is important for this higher-risk patient with IBD group.

For older patients with a previous history of malignancy, the risk of cancer recurrence seems to be highest within the first 2 years after cancer treatment.[48] For the patients with IBD newly in remission from cancer, initiating thiopurine therapy may not be recommended by oncologists, although data from the CESAME cohort reported no significant differences in new or recurrent cancer rates among thiopurine treated and unexposed patients followed for a median of 3 years.[49] For patients with newly diagnosed cancers receiving treatment, oncologists may recommend discontinuation of thiopurines because of concerns about increasing bone marrow suppression risk and infection while on conventional chemotherapy.[50] However, the approach to IBD management in the setting of cancer largely depends on the degree of IBD activity, the choice of chemotherapeutic regimen, and the risks of IBD therapy, not only relating to continued cancer treatments but also for the cancer-treated older patient. Thus, a multidisciplinary approach involving the gastroenterologist and oncologist is advised before initiating or discontinuing therapy.

Biological Treatment in the Elderly

Among the treatment options currently available for moderate to severe IBD, the anti-TNF agents have shown efficacy to induce and maintain remission as well as lead to mucosal healing. However, the safety and efficacy of the anti-TNF agents for the treatment of the older patient with IBD have not been well established, because many of these older patients were excluded from the randomized controlled trials. An Italian study comparing clinical remission rates among patients older than 65 years treated with biologics versus patients younger than 65 years found no significant differences in clinical remission rates based on subjective symptom scores. However, the older biologic-treated patients were more susceptible to AEs, including serious infections, with a reported 10% mortality.[51] Desai and colleagues[52] reported lower 6-month response rates to anti-TNF therapy among older patients with IBD (61%) compared with younger patients (83%). The older patients with IBD were also 4 times more likely to discontinue anti-TNF therapy compared with younger patients, with 70% of older patients stopping their anti-TNF therapy at 24 months because of lack of efficacy or AEs. In addition, 22% of older patients treated with anti-TNF experienced infections, and 32% of patients had other anti-TNF–associated AEs. Similar rates of medication discontinuation because of lack of therapeutic efficacy or AEs have also been reported among older patients with rheumatoid arthritis.[53,54]

Older patients with IBD may also have comorbidities that preclude the use of anti-TNF agents. Anti-TNF agents should not be administered to patients with an established diagnosis of multiple sclerosis and should be given with caution in the setting of other demyelinating disorders.[55] Etanercept and infliximab (IFX) were studied as potential treatments for congestive heart failure (CHF). These studies were terminated early because of lack of efficacy and also, more importantly, because of serious AEs occurring among patients treated with anti-TNF, including increased mortality and CHF exacerbation.[56,57] Therefore, patients with class III or IV CHF should not be treated with anti-TNF agents, whereas patients with class I or II CHF may be administered anti-TNF therapies with caution.[55,56] Before prescribing anti-TNF agents to older patients with cardiac morbidity, it may be appropriate to consider cardiac consultation or obtain updated cardiac testing. For patients with preexisting interstitial lung disease, anti-TNF therapy should be given with caution, with routine monitoring of pulmonary function and discontinuation of therapy with worsened respiratory status.[55] Although there are only limited data looking at the impact of anti-TNF therapy among former smokers and patients with chronic obstructive pulmonary disease (COPD), a small study of patients with COPD who were treated with IFX found a nonsignificant increase in lung cancer among IFX-treated patients (9 cases out of 157 IFX-treated patients) compared with placebo (1 case out of 77 patients).[58] For patients with a history of malignancy, particularly if the malignancy was greater than 5 years previously, anti-TNF therapy may not be contraindicated if the cancer is in remission. However, anti-TNF use in the setting of current or recent malignancy should be reserved for moderate to severe disease activity that is not responsive to corticosteroids after consultation with oncology, because of the potential risk of recurrent malignancy or adverse reactions.[50]

Although the older patient with IBD may be more susceptible to AEs of anti-TNF therapy, additional longitudinal studies are needed to determine the efficacy and safety of these medications in clinical practice. Many of the studies reporting increased anti-TNF–related complications were among older patients with IBD maintained on chronic steroids in combination with the biological therapies or with prolonged disease activity before medication initiation. Therefore, the AEs attributed to the anti-TNFs may also reflect sequelae of prolonged disease activity and steroid-associated AEs. It is possible that optimization of disease activity with earlier initiation of anti-TNF therapies before the development of features more indicative of active disease such as anemia, malnutrition, or weight loss, which are also associated with increased AE risk among older patients with IBD, could yield better outcomes.

Medication Utilization Among Elderly Patients with IBD

Compared with prescribing to younger patients with IBD, practitioners tend to prescribe thiopurines or biologics less often to older patients with IBD. For patients with late-onset IBD, representing approximately 10% to 15% of new diagnoses annually, this finding may be a reflection of a more mild disease course compared with younger patients at the time of diagnosis.[1,59] Late-onset IBD tends to present as UC or colonic CD, with low rates of disease progression to penetrating or stricturing disease, which are associated with greater disease-related complications.[60] Charpentier and colleagues[60] described the natural history of 841 newly diagnosed older patients with IBD within the EPIMAD registry in France. These late-onset patients with IBD were treated primarily with 5-ASA and corticosteroids, with only 16% of patients receiving thiopurines and 7% of patients prescribed biologics. In another study of patients with late-onset UC, although 82% of patients had moderate to severe symptoms at diagnosis, they were primarily treated with corticosteroids (68%) and 5-ASAs (96%). At 1 year, 64% of patients were in a steroid-free remission, maintained primarily on 5-ASAs, with only 6% of patients requiring IFX and 29% of patients prescribed immunomodulators. However, almost 30% of the patients with late-onset IBD studied were still symptomatic at 1 year with moderate to severe disease activity.[61] Similarly, within the EPIMAD registry, approximately 20% of steroid-treated older patients with IBD were steroid dependent at 1 year after diagnosis.[60] These data suggest that although the most patients with late-onset IBD may have mild disease activity controlled with 5-ASA agents, a significant percentage of older patients with newly diagnosed IBD have more active disease, warranting escalation of therapy to involve more potent immunosuppression.

For patients with IBD with moderate to severe symptoms, corticosteroids and anti-TNF agents are given to induce remission, whereas thiopurines and anti-TNFs either alone or in combination are used to maintain remission. However, these agents seem to be underused for the older patient with IBD. A study looking at prescribing patterns among elderly patients with IBD in the United States[62] reported that 20% to 36% of patients were prescribed oral corticosteroids during the 6-year study period, whereas only 9% to 28% of patients received thiopurines and 1% to 15% of patients received anti-TNF therapies. Another study of 393 geriatric patients with IBD[63] reported that 32% of patients were taking corticosteroids as a maintenance IBD medication defined as greater than 6 months of continued use with no documentation of potential steroid-sparing exit strategies. Within this study cohort, only 7% of patients were maintained on immunomodulators and only 3% received anti-TNFs.

The relative underprescribing of thiopurines and biologics within the older patient with IBD cohort may reflect prescribers' concerns about the potential AEs of immunosuppression, such as serious infection and malignancy, outweighing the potential steroid-sparing benefits with respect to IBD activity. However, the high percentage of steroid use among older patients with IBD is concerning and may be responsible for some of the poorer clinical outcomes. Greater than 25% of IBD-associated hospitalizations occur within the oldest age group, with associated increased lengths of stay, costs of care, and in-hospital mortality. The primary indications for hospitalization reflect not only disease activity but the inability of the older patients to handle the burden of disease, with gastrointestinal bleeding, dehydration, malnutrition, anemia, and electrolyte disturbances noted as common indications for admission.[64] Appropriate prescribing of steroid-sparing IBD therapies relative to disease severity earlier during the clinical course may prevent these hospitalizations related to disease activity rather than continuing medications such as 5-ASAs, which have little role for moderate to severe symptoms in CD or maintenance steroids.

Polypharmacy and the Older Patient with IBD

Polypharmacy is another major factor to consider in the management of the older patient with IBD. Increasing numbers of routine medications lead to greater risks of drug interactions, prescribing cascades, and decreased adherence. Among patients with IBD aged 65 years and older, patients with CD were taking an average of 10 routine medications and patients with UC were taking an average of 9 routine medications. Almost half of these older patients with IBD (46%) had severe polypharmacy, defined as greater than 10 routine medications. Nearly two-thirds of these patients had at least 1 drug-drug interaction involving 1 of the IBD medications, and 26% of patients had a major drug interaction with their IBD medications.[65] Risk factors associated with increased polypharmacy among this geriatric IBD cohort included increased comorbidity and chronic steroid use.[65] Another study of 291 patients with IBD[66] reported that 50% of patients with CD had major polypharmacy, defined as greater than 5 routine medications, and increasing polypharmacy was associated with higher disease activity scores and lower quality-of-life scores. Many older Americans also take multiple vitamins, minerals, and other over-the-counter supplements, which increase daily pill burden.[5] Careful review of updated medication lists at each office visit, with elimination of unnecessary agents, may help decrease polypharmacy and associated drug interactions, particularly because many older patients see multiple specialists to manage their comorbidities. Avoidance of inappropriate medications, particularly narcotic, sedative, and anticholinergic agents, may also decrease the risk of medication-associated complications.[67]

SUMMARY

Management of the older patient with IBD is more nuanced than younger patients, reflecting the added complexities associated with aging. Although mucosal healing and deep remission are goals of IBD therapy, the treatment paradigms may need to be modified for older patients with IBD. Medical decision making for the older patient with IBD extends beyond disease-related risks and benefits of treatments to also include considerations of comorbidity, functional status, and ability to handle disease burden. For the fit older patient with IBD, the management is largely similar to the younger patient; however, for the frail older patient with IBD, conventional treatment algorithms may increase risk of AEs, hospitalizations, or mortality.[68]

Simplified medication regimens are best for the older patients with IBD, especially considering the higher rates of polypharmacy and increased potential for medication interactions. Updated medication lists containing prescription as well as over-the-counter medications and supplements should be provided to all members of the care team, with routine checks performed for drug interaction. Decreasing daily pill burden, reducing dosing frequencies, and eliminating unnecessary medications may improve adherence to therapies. Establishing appropriate family or home health support to help organize medications, with clear labeling, may help overcome issues relating to visual impairment and inability to discriminate the types of medication, which may lead to erroneous consumption of medications.

With respect to IBD-specific treatments, finite end points to steroid-based therapies should be defined at the start of therapy, with a planned exit strategy to avoid prolonged steroid courses. Earlier recognition of flares, with more frequent outpatient visits, may allow for earlier initiation of immunomodulators or biologics for moderate to severe disease activity on a case-by-case basis. However, given the increased risk of AEs associated with immunosuppressive therapies, extended trials of immunosuppression should be avoided if it is ineffective. If medications have not shown efficacy within the specified induction window at conventional dosing, the benefit of prolonged or increased dosing may not outweigh the risk. To decrease risk of serious infections, fractures, and malignancy related to medical therapy, health care maintenance should be updated routinely, including vaccinations, bone densitometry, dental and vision examinations, and age-appropriate cancer screening. With coordinated care and heightened monitoring of the older patient with IBD, the age-appropriate balance of inflammatory disease control and patient safety may be achieved.

REFERENCES

1. Khalili H, Huang ES, Ananthakrishnan AN, et al. Geographical variation and incidence of inflammatory bowel disease among US women. Gut 2012;61:1686–92.
2. Klotz U. Pharmacokinetics and drug metabolism in the elderly. Drug Metab Rev 2009;41:67–76.
3. Tinetti ME, Bogardus ST Jr, Agostini JV. Potential pitfalls of disease-specific guidelines for patients with multiple conditions. N Engl J Med 2004;351:2870–4.
4. Gurwitz JH, Field TS, Harrold LR, et al. Incidence and preventability of adverse drug events among older persons in the ambulatory setting. JAMA 2003;289:1107–16.
5. Qato DM, Alexander GC, Conti RM, et al. Use of prescription and over-the-counter medications and dietary supplements among older adults in the United States. JAMA 2008;300:2867–78.

6. Kaufman DW, Kelly JP, Rosenberg L, et al. Recent patterns of medication use in the ambulatory adult population of the United States: the Slone survey. JAMA 2002;287:337–44.

7. Rochon PA, Gurwitz JH. Optimising drug treatment for elderly people: the prescribing cascade. BMJ 1997;315:1096–9.

8. Pineton de Chambrun G, Peyrin-Biroulet L, Lemann M, et al. Clinical implications of mucosal healing for the management of IBD. Nat Rev Gastroenterol Hepatol 2010;7:15–29.

9. D'Haens G, Baert F, van Assche G, et al. Early combined immunosuppression or conventional management in patients with newly diagnosed Crohn's disease: an open randomised trial. Lancet 2008;371:660–7.

10. Colombel JF, Sandborn WJ, Reinisch W, et al. Infliximab, azathioprine, or combination therapy for Crohn's disease. N Engl J Med 2010;362:1383–95.

11. Lichtenstein GR, Yan S, Bala M, et al. Infliximab maintenance treatment reduces hospitalizations, surgeries, and procedures in fistulizing Crohn's disease. Gastroenterology 2005;128:862–9.

12. Lichtenstein GR, Feagan BG, Cohen RD, et al. Serious infection and mortality in patients with Crohn's disease: more than 5 years of follow-up in the TREAT registry. Am J Gastroenterol 2012;107:1409–22.

13. Tourner M, Loftus EV, Harmsen WS, et al. Risk factors for opportunistic infections in patients with inflammatory bowel disease. Gastroenterology 2008;134:929–36.

14. Grijalva CG, Chen L, Delzell E, et al. Initiation of tumor necrosis factor-alpha antagonists and the risk of hospitalization for infection in patients with autoimmune diseases. JAMA 2011;306:2331–9.

15. Ha CY, Katz S. Clinical outcomes and management of inflammatory bowel disease in the older patient. Curr Gastroenterol Rep 2013;15:310–7.

16. Lichtenstein GR, Feagan BG, Cohen RD, et al. Serious infectious and mortality in association with therapies for Crohn's disease: TREAT registry. Clin Gastroenterol Hepatol 2006;4:621–30.

17. Castle SC. Clinical relevance of age-related immune dysfunction. Clin Infect Dis 2000;31:578–85.

18. Pawelec G. Immunosenescence: impact in the young as well as the old? Mech Ageing Dev 1999;108:1–7.

19. Cucchiara S, Iebba V, Conte MP, et al. The microbiota in inflammatory bowel disease in different age groups. Dig Dis 2009;27:252–8.

20. Ananthakrishnan AN, McGinley EL, Binion DG. Excess hospitalisation burden associated with *Clostridium difficile* in patients with inflammatory bowel disease. Gut 2008;57:205–10.

21. Ananthakrishnan AN, McGinley EL. Infection-related hospitalizations are associated with increased mortality in patients with inflammatory bowel diseases. J Crohns Colitis 2013;7:107–12.

22. Katz S, Pardi DS. Inflammatory bowel disease of the elderly: frequently asked questions (FAQs). Am J Gastroenterol 2011;106:1889–97.

23. Lichtenstein GR, Hanauer SB, Sandborn WJ. Management of Crohn's disease in adults. Am J Gastroenterol 2009;104:465–83.

24. Kornbluth A, Sachar DB. Ulcerative colitis practice guidelines in adults: American College Of Gastroenterology, Practice Parameters Committee. Am J Gastroenterol 2010;105:501–23.

25. Ford AC, Khan KJ, Sandborn WJ, et al. Once-daily dosing vs. conventional dosing schedule of mesalamine and relapse of quiescent ulcerative colitis: systematic review and meta-analysis. Am J Gastroenterol 2011;106:2070–7.

26. Kane SV, Sumner M, Solomon D, et al. Twelve-month persistency with oral 5-aminosalicylic acid therapy for ulcerative colitis: results from a large pharmacy prescriptions database. Dig Dis Sci 2011;56:3463–70.
27. Kapur KC, Williams GT, Allison MC. Mesalazine induced exacerbation of ulcerative colitis. Gut 1995;37:838–9.
28. Regueiro M, Loftus EV Jr, Steinhart AH, et al. Medical management of left-sided ulcerative colitis and ulcerative proctitis: critical evaluation of therapeutic trials. Inflamm Bowel Dis 2006;12:979–94.
29. Safdi M, DeMicco M, Sninsky C, et al. A double-blind comparison of oral versus rectal mesalamine versus combination therapy in the treatment of distal ulcerative colitis. Am J Gastroenterol 1997;92:1867–71.
30. Marshall JK, Thabane M, Steinhart AH, et al. Rectal 5-aminosalicylic acid for induction of remission in ulcerative colitis. Cochrane Database Syst Rev 2010;(1):CD004115.
31. Rao SS. Diagnosis and management of fecal incontinence. American College of Gastroenterology Practice Parameters Committee. Am J Gastroenterol 2004;99: 1585–604.
32. Boyle DJ, Knowles CH, Murphy J, et al. The effects of age and childbirth on anal sphincter function and morphology in 999 symptomatic female patients with colorectal dysfunction. Dis Colon Rectum 2012;55:286–93.
33. Gisbert JP, Gonzalez-Lama Y, Mate J. 5-Aminosalicylates and renal function in inflammatory bowel disease: a systematic review. Inflamm Bowel Dis 2007;13: 629–38.
34. So K, Bewshea CM, Heap GA, et al. 5-Aminosalicylate (5-ASA) induced nephrotoxicity in inflammatory bowel disease. Gastroenterology 2013;144:S112.
35. Thomas TP. The complications of systemic corticosteroid therapy in the elderly. A retrospective study. Gerontology 1984;30:60–5.
36. Akerkar GA, Peppercorn MA, Hamel MB, et al. Corticosteroid-associated complications in elderly Crohn's disease patients. Am J Gastroenterol 1997;92:461–4.
37. Ananthakrishnan AN, McGinley EL, Binion DG, et al. Fracture-associated hospitalizations in patients with inflammatory bowel disease. Dig Dis Sci 2011;56: 176–82.
38. Bernstein CN. Osteoporosis and other complications of inflammatory bowel disease. Curr Opin Gastroenterol 2002;18:428–34.
39. Moscandrew M, Mahadevan U, Kane S. General health maintenance in IBD. Inflamm Bowel Dis 2009;15:1399–409.
40. Timmer A, McDonald JW, Macdonald JK. Azathioprine and 6-mercaptopurine for maintenance of remission in ulcerative colitis. Cochrane Database Syst Rev 2007;(1):CD000478.
41. Prefontaine E, Macdonald JK, Sutherland LR. Azathioprine or 6-mercaptopurine for induction of remission in Crohn's disease. Cochrane Database Syst Rev 2009;(4):CD000545.
42. Irving PM, Shanahan F, Rampton DS. Drug interactions in inflammatory bowel disease. Am J Gastroenterol 2008;103:207–19.
43. Bermejo F, Gisbert JP. Usefulness of salicylate and thiopurine coprescription in steroid-dependent ulcerative colitis and withdrawal strategies. Ther Adv Chronic Dis 2010;1:107–14.
44. Khan N, Abbas A, Lichtenstein GR, et al. Risk of lymphoma in patients with ulcerative colitis treated with thiopurines - a nationwide retrospective cohort study. Gastroenterology 2013. http://dx.doi.org/10.1053/j.gastro.2013.07.035.

45. Beaugerie L, Brousse N, Bouvier AM, et al. Lymphoproliferative disorders in patients receiving thiopurines for inflammatory bowel disease: a prospective observational cohort study. Lancet 2009;374:1617–25.
46. Long MD, Martin CF, Pipkin CA, et al. Risk of melanoma and nonmelanoma skin cancer among patients with inflammatory bowel disease. Gastroenterology 2012;143:390–9.
47. Peyrin-Biroulet L, Khosrotehrani K, Carrat F, et al. Increased risk for nonmelanoma skin cancers in patients who receive thiopurines for inflammatory bowel disease. Gastroenterology 2011;141:1621–8.
48. Penn I. Evaluation of transplant candidates with pre-existing malignancies. Ann Transplant 1997;2:14–7.
49. Beaugerie L, Carrat F, Chevaux JB, et al. Risk of subsequent cancer under immunosuppressive therapy in patients with inflammatory bowel disease and prior cancer: data from the CESAME prospective observational cohort. Gastroenterology 2012;142:S122.
50. Bernheim O, Colombel JF, Ullman TA, et al. The management of immunosuppression in patients with inflammatory bowel disease and cancer. Gut 2013; 62(11):1523–8. http://dx.doi.org/10.1136/gutjnl-2013-305300.
51. Cottone M, Kohn A, Daperno M, et al. Age is a risk factor for severe infections and mortality in patients given anti-tumor necrosis factor therapy for inflammatory bowel disease. Clin Gastroenterol Hepatol 2010;9:30–5.
52. Desai A, Zator ZA, de Silva P, et al. Older age is associated with higher rate of discontinuation of anti-TNF therapy in patients with inflammatory bowel disease. Inflamm Bowel Dis 2013;19(2):309–15. http://dx.doi.org/10.1002/ibd.23026.
53. Tran S, Hooker RS, Cipher DJ, et al. Patterns of biologic agent use in older males with inflammatory diseases: an institution-focused, observational postmarketing study. Drugs Aging 2009;26:607–15.
54. Oei HB, Hooker RS, Cipher DJ, et al. High rates of stopping or switching biological medications in veterans with rheumatoid arthritis. Clin Exp Rheumatol 2009; 27:926–34.
55. Ding T, Ledingham J, Luqmani R, et al. BSR and BHPR rheumatoid arthritis guidelines on safety of anti-TNF therapies. Rheumatology 2010;49:2217–9.
56. Chung ES, Packer M, Lo KH, et al. Randomized, double-blind, placebo-controlled, pilot trial of infliximab, a chimeric monoclonal antibody to tumor necrosis factor-alpha, in patients with moderate-to-severe heart failure: results of the anti-TNF Therapy Against Congestive Heart Failure (ATTACH) trial. Circulation 2003;107:3133–40.
57. Mann DL, McMurray JJ, Packer M, et al. Targeted anticytokine therapy in patients with chronic heart failure: results of the Randomized Etanercept Worldwide Evaluation (RENEWAL). Circulation 2004;109:1594–602.
58. Rennard SI, Fogarty C, Kelsen S, et al. The safety and efficacy of infliximab in moderate to severe chronic obstructive pulmonary disease. Am J Respir Crit Care Med 2007;175:926–34.
59. Loftus CG, Loftus EV Jr, Harmsen WS, et al. Update on the incidence and prevalence of Crohn's disease and ulcerative colitis in Olmsted County, Minnesota, 1940-2000. Inflamm Bowel Dis 2007;13:254–61.
60. Charpentier C, Salleron J, Savoye G, et al. Natural history of elderly-onset inflammatory bowel disease: a population-based cohort study. Gut 2013. http://dx.doi.org/10.1136/gutjnl-2012-303864.

61. Ha CY, Newberry RD, Stone CD, et al. Patients with late-adult-onset ulcerative colitis have better outcomes than those with early onset disease. Clin Gastroenterol Hepatol 2010;8:682–7.

62. Benchimol EI, Cook SF, Erichsen R, et al. International variation in medication prescription rates among elderly patients with inflammatory bowel disease. J Crohns Colitis 2012;7(11):878–89. http://dx.doi.org/10.1016/j.crohns.2012.09.001.

63. Juneja M, Baidoo L, Schwartz MB, et al. Geriatric inflammatory bowel disease: phenotypic presentation, treatment patterns, nutritional status, outcomes, and comorbidity. Dig Dis Sci 2012;57:2408–15.

64. Ananthakrishnan AN, McGinley EL, Binion DG. Inflammatory bowel disease in the elderly is associated with worse outcomes: a national study of hospitalizations. Inflamm Bowel Dis 2009;15:182–9.

65. Parian A, Ha C. Severe polypharmacy and major medication interactions are associated with increasing age and comorbidity among inflammatory bowel disease patients. Gastroenterology 2013;144:S11.

66. Cross RK, Wilson KT, Binion DG. Polypharmacy and Crohn's disease. Aliment Pharmacol Ther 2005;21:1211–6.

67. American Geriatrics Society 2012 Beers Criteria Update Expert Panel. American Geriatrics Society updated Beers Criteria for potentially inappropriate medication use in older adults. J Am Geriatr Soc 2012;60:616–31.

68. Katz S, Surawicz C, Pardi DS. Management of the elderly patients with inflammatory bowel disease: practical considerations. Inflamm Bowel Dis 2013;19:2257–72.

Clostridium difficile Infection in the Elderly

Jonathan M. Keller, MD[a], Christina M. Surawicz, MD[b],*

KEYWORDS

- Antibiotic-associated diarrhea • *Clostridium difficile* • Elderly

KEY POINTS

- *Clostridium difficile* infection (CDI) is an increasingly prevalent disease that disproportionately affects elderly populations.
- Rates of severe disease, medical complications, and mortality are higher for older patients.
- CDI is preventable primarily through prudent antibiotic use and infection-control measures.
- The cornerstone of CDI therapy remains antibiotic treatment, although several novel interventions are emerging as effective management regimens.

INTRODUCTION

Clostridium difficile infection (CDI) is the most common cause of nosocomial diarrhea in the industrialized world.[1,2] In some areas, such the Southern United States, *C difficile* have surpassed the infection rate of other health care–associated infections, such as methicillin-resistant *Staphylococcus aureus*.[3] It is also the most common infectious cause of acute diarrhea in nursing homes, accounting for at least one-quarter of cases.[4,5]

The incidence and mortality of CDI has significantly increased over the past decade. According to nationwide data from the Agency for Healthcare Research and Quality, the number of hospital stays related to CDI increased 300% between 1993 and 2008, although this number seemed to plateau in 2009 around 337,000 stays, representing nearly 1% of all hospitalizations.[6] CDI also carried a nearly five-fold increased risk of mortality and patients were hospitalized 8 days longer than average, with an estimated economic burden of $500 million annually.[7] This increased disease

[a] Department of Medicine, University of Washington Medical Center, 1959 Northeast Pacific Street, Box 356421, Seattle, WA 98195, USA; [b] Division of Gastroenterology, Harborview Medical Center, University of Washington School of Medicine, 325 9th Avenue, Box 359773, Seattle, WA 98104, USA
* Corresponding author.
E-mail address: surawicz@u.washington.edu

Clin Geriatr Med 30 (2014) 79–93
http://dx.doi.org/10.1016/j.cger.2013.10.008
0749-0690/14/$ – see front matter © 2014 Elsevier Inc. All rights reserved.

geriatric.theclinics.com

burden is partly caused by development of a hyperviruent strain, commonly known as BI/NAP1/027. This ribotype is associated with fluoroquinolone resistance and is responsible for outbreaks of severe and often fatal colitis in North America and Europe, especially in elderly patients.[8–10]

CDI disproportionately affects older adults, with those 65 and older accounting for most disease morbidity and mortality.[11] Hospital stays related to C difficile occurred at a rate of 1089 per 100,000 for patients ages 85 and older, more than double that of the next age cohort (**Fig. 1**).[6] In 2008, C difficile ranked as the 18th leading cause of death for the population aged 65 and older, and approximately 92% of deaths from C difficile occurred in people aged 65 and older.[12] In addition, geriatric populations are more likely to develop sequelae from CDI, including severe disease with end-organ complications and recurrent infections.[13]

CLINICAL OVERVIEW

C difficile is an anaerobic gram-positive bacillus that is spore-forming and toxin-producing,[14] initially discovered to be a causative agent of pseudomembranous colitis in 1978.[15] The spore form of the organism can live for long periods of time in relatively harsh environments, facilitating persistence in such locations as hospitals and health care facilities. Transmission occurs through the fecal-oral route, whereupon reaching the colon ingested spores can germinate into a metabolically active vegetative state and subsequently lead to clinical disease.

Alteration of the normal intestinal microbiome, through antibiotic use for example, is thought to facilitate C difficile overgrowth and subsequent disease.[16] The pathogenic effects are primarily derived from the elaboration of two large-molecular-weight exotoxins, toxin A and the more potent toxin B. The exotoxins induce mucosal inflammation and secretory diarrhea through disruption of the intestinal epithelial cytoskeleton and tight junctions.[17]

The clinical manifestations of C difficile range from asymptomatic carriage, to mild diarrhea, to colitis, to pseudomembranous colitis with toxic megacolon (**Fig. 2**). Asymptomatic colonic infection can occur with toxigenic and nontoxigenic strains,[18] suggesting host-specific factors play an important role in disease manifestation. Studies have correlated the strength of humoral immune responses to C difficile toxins to disease severity,[19,20] a defense mechanism that deteriorates with age.[21]

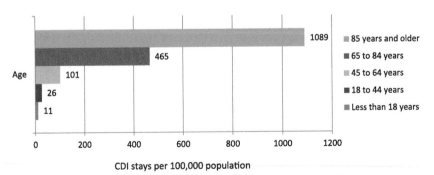

Fig. 1. Rate of principal and secondary diagnosis of CDI stays per 100,000 population by age group, 2009. (*Data from* Lucado J, Gould C, Elixhauser A. *Clostridium difficile* infections (CDI) in hospital stays. Healthcare Cost and Utilization Project, Agency for Healthcare Research and Quality Statistical Brief #124 2009.)

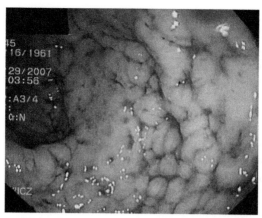

Fig. 2. Confluent pseudomembranes in a patient with *Clostridium difficile* colitis. (*From* Knight CL, Surawicz CM. *Clostridium difficile* infection. Med Clin North Am 2013;97:526; with permission.)

Mild disease consists of diarrhea as the only symptom, whereas moderate disease includes additional signs or symptoms not meeting criteria for severe or complicated CDI, such as abdominal cramping. For more severe disease, the 2013 American College of Gastroenterology guidelines[22] recommend following three independent risk factors determined by multivariate analysis to predict severe disease: (1) abdominal distention, (2) elevated white blood cell count, and (3) hypoalbuminemia. Severe disease is defined as hypoalbuminemia less than 3 g/dL and either white blood cell count greater than 15,000 cells/mm^3 or abdominal tenderness without criteria of complicated disease. Severe and complicated disease includes CDI with at least one of the following: admission to the intensive care unit, hypotension with or without vasopressor support, fever greater than or equal to 38.5°C, ileus, significant abdominal distention, mental status changes, white blood cell count greater than 35,000 cells/mm^3 or less than 2000 cells/mm^3, lactate greater than 2.2 mmol/L, or any evidence of end organ failure.

There are no data to suggest disease presentation is uniformly or significantly different in elderly patients, other than the higher rates of advanced disease and clinical complications previously described. One possible exception is *C difficile* enteritis involving the small bowel in patients without inflammatory bowel disease, which is exceedingly rare, but almost exclusively seen in elderly patients.[23]

RISK FACTORS

The most important risk factors for CDI are advanced age, and exposure to antibiotics and to health care environments, although myriad other factors play a role in the incidence and severity of disease (**Table 1**).

Age

Advanced age is a well-demonstrated risk factor for CDI in epidemiologic studies, with the increased risk burden thought to begin at age 65.[24] A recent cohort study reviewing CDI across six Canadian hospitals over 15 months found that for each year of age, the risk of health care–acquired CDI increases by 2%.[25] The reason for this is likely multifactorial related primarily to prevalent comorbid illnesses, increased pharmaceutical use including antibiotics, and increased exposure to health care

Table 1
Risk factors for *Clostridium difficile* infection in the elderly

Risk Factor	Important Features
Age	Risk increases after age 65 by 2% per year of age Intestinal flora changes with age and may predispose to infection Humoral immune defenses are less robust in the elderly
Antibiotics	Alters intestinal flora and allows for *C difficile* overgrowth Most commonly implicated antibiotics are clindamycin, aminopenicillins, second- and third-generation cephalosporins and fluoroquinolones Risk for CDI is highest 2 wk after antibiotic therapy, but persists for 3 mo Antibiotic stewardship programs reduce CDI rates
Health care exposures	Asymptomatic carriage of *C difficile* occurs in 20%–30% of hospitalized patients and up to 50% of residents at long-term care facilities Risk of CDI in inpatients increases with longer durations of stay and more antibiotic administration Most CDI cases in long-term care facilities occur within 30 d of admission
Other factors	Increased number of comorbidities is associated with CDI Antisecretory agents, such as proton-pump inhibitors, likely predispose to CDI

environments. Not every patient who acquires *C difficile*, however, manifests symptomatic disease, suggesting there are additional host and microenvironment factors that influence disease phenotype.

Intestinal flora is well known to change with age, and may increase susceptibility to *C difficile* colonization. Microbiologic studies have demonstrated the marked difference of microbiotas of elderly patients with CDI compared with those in healthy elderly subjects, with fewer competing anaerobes, such as *Bacteroides* and *Bifidobacterium*,[26] confirmed in subsequent studies.[27,28] Further studies are needed, however, to elucidate the importance of microbiota dysbiosis and clinical implications, such as directed therapeutic probiotic supplementation.

Particular attention has been directed toward the impaired immune responses of the elderly that occur naturally with aging, suggesting these patients are less able to mount an immune response to infection.[29,30] This phenomenon of immunosenescence has been purported as a potential mechanism for more frequent and severe *C difficile*–associated disease in elderly patients. Elevated antitoxin immunoglobulins have been shown to favorably affect outcomes of *C difficile* colonization,[20] shorten disease duration,[31] and influence risk of recurrence.[19] A recent prospective cohort study more specifically demonstrated correlation between low systemic antitoxin A IgG levels and mortality during severe CDI.[32] Impaired humoral response was independent of age in this particular study, although most of the study population was elderly and the functional capacity of the antitoxin IgG was not investigated.

Antibiotics

Alteration of the normal intestinal flora through antibiotic exposure is the major modifiable risk factor for developing CDI. The reduction of competing microbiota allows for overgrowth of either indigenous *C difficile* organisms or novel infection. Essentially all antibiotics carry a risk of CDI, although the most frequently implicated are clindamycin, aminopenicillins, and second- or third- generation cephalosporins.[33] Fluoroquinolone-associated CDI is becoming increasingly prevalent with the emergence of the BI/NAP1/027 *C difficile* strain noted for its reduced susceptibility to fluoroquinolone antibiotics and responsible for several outbreaks in the United States, Canada, and Europe primarily affecting older patients.[34]

The risk for CDI is most prominent in the first 2 weeks of antibiotic therapy, but persists up to 3 months after discontinuation of the drug.[35] The risk also seems to be cumulative, because the greater the number of antimicrobials used and the longer the duration of treatment, the higher the conferred risk of *C difficile* acquisition.[36] This poses particular concern for elderly people with higher burdens of illness that prompt more frequent antibiotic use. Although antibiotic stewardship programs are being developed throughout the world to more judiciously implement therapeutic antimicrobial use, there is no uniform programmatic system for which to monitor and guide its use.[37,38]

Hospitalization and Long-term Care Facilities

Although the incidence of community-acquired CDI is increasing,[39] most infections result after exposure to health care environments, where *C difficile* spores are more prevalent.[40] Nearly 3% of asymptomatic adults are colonized with *C difficile*,[41] dramatically increasing to 20% to 30% carriage rate in hospitalized patients[42] and up to 50% of patients residing in long-term care facilities.[43] There is growing evidence suggesting asymptomatic carriers of *C difficile* far outnumbering the cases of symptomatic diarrheal illness significantly contribute to transmission in hospitals.[44] The risk of CDI increases with longer durations of hospitalization[45] and admission to a room where the prior occupant suffered from CDI.[46]

Studies have shown up to 40% to 50% of CDI cases were acquired in long-term care facilities.[47,48] In some areas, however, most CDI in long-term care facilities occurred within 30 days of admission and predominantly in patients undergoing subacute rehabilitation.[49] These data suggest *C difficile* disease burden may be overestimated for chronic care facilities and more extensive studies are needed to determine what proportion of these cases are, in fact, hospital-acquired.

Other Factors

There are several additional factors associated with CDI. Patients with more comorbid conditions in general are more susceptible to CDI. The presence of inflammatory bowel disease is specifically linked to more frequent and severe disease with poorer clinical outcomes,[50] and the American College of Gastroenterology strongly recommends testing for CDI for all patients with inflammatory bowel disease presenting with a flare.[22] Other associations with CDI include immunosuppression following transplantation,[51,52] tube feeding,[53] chronic liver disease,[54] chronic kidney disease,[55] and gastrointestinal surgery,[56] all increasingly common in elderly populations.

Much attention has been directed toward antisecretory agents, which purportedly predispose to CDI by limiting natural sterilization[57] and altering intestinal flora.[58] A recent systematic review confirmed earlier findings that proton-pump inhibitor use is associated with incident and recurrent CDI, with odds ratios of 1.74 and 2.51, respectively.[59] This translates into an estimated additional 15 cases of CDI for every 1000 hospital inpatients resulting from proton-pump inhibitor use. There also seems to be a synergistic effect with antibiotics, beyond that of either medication class alone. Histamine$_2$-receptor antagonists are less harmful than proton-pump inhibitors but still carry a risk. The need for antisecretory pharmaceuticals and the duration of use, especially in elderly patients at higher risk of CDI, should be critically evaluated on a continual basis. Up to 63% of patients who developed CDI while on a proton-pump inhibitor did not have a valid indication for acid-suppression therapy.[60]

Use of antidepressants has been associated with CDI as an ancillary finding in cohort studies.[61] More recent observational studies have identified a link among

CDI, major depression, and particular antidepressants,[62] but this has yet to be evaluated in a prospective randomized fashion.

Epidemiologic and case-control studies suggest that statin medications decrease the risk of CDI,[63,64] presumably because of the pleiotropic anti-inflammatory properties but a true causal relationship has not been determined.

MANAGEMENT STRATEGIES

The management of CDI depends on the severity of disease and several patient factors. The most recent American College of Gastroenterology guidelines[22] augment the Infectious Disease Society of America and Society for Healthcare Epidemiology of America treatment guidelines from 2010[65] and are outlined below. The mainstay of treatment remains antibiotic treatment with metronidazole and vancomycin, although several novel treatment strategies are under development with promising results (**Table 2**).

Diagnosis

Diagnosis of CDI is usually made by detection of C difficile toxins in the stool, although no test is perfect. The gold standard laboratory reference tests are toxigenic culture (strains that do not product toxin are not pathogenic) and tissue culture assay for toxin B. Both tests are expensive and take several days for results and thus are not practical for clinical care. Enzyme immunoassay tests for toxins A and B were

Table 2
Treatment of CDI based on 2013 American College of Gastroenterology recommendations

Category	Definition	Recommendation
Mild-Moderate	Diarrhea with additional symptoms not meeting criteria for severe or complicated disease	Metronidazole 500 mg 3×/d for 10 d
Severe	Albumin <3 g/dL and either white blood cell count >15,000 cells/mm^3 or abdominal tenderness	Vancomycin 125 mg po 4×/d for 10 d
Complicated	Any of the following criteria met: White blood cell count >35,000 cells/mm^3 or <2000 cells/mm^3 Lactate >2.2 mmol/L Admission to the intensive care unit Hypotension with or without vasopressor support Fever ≥38.5°C Ileus or abdominal distention Mental status changes End organ failure	Vancomycin 500 mg 4×/d po or by nasogastric tube plus intravenous metronidazole 500 mg 3×/d; if complete ileus, vancomycin can be given rectally
First recurrence		Treat like first episode
Second recurrence		Vancomycin taper and pulse: 125 mg po 4x/d for 10 d then 125 mg a day every 3 d for 10 more doses
Third or more recurrence		Consider fecal microbiota transplant

Data from Surawicz CM, Brandt LJ, Binion DG, et al. Guidelines for diagnosis, treatment, and prevention of *Clostridium difficile* infections. Am J Gastroenterol 2013;108:478–98; [quiz: 499].

widely used until recently, because they are rapid and relatively inexpensive. However, they have poor sensitivity; a negative test in a patient with a high likelihood of CDI should not preclude the start of empiric therapy. In many academic centers, enzyme immunoassay tests are rapidly being replaced by nucleic acid amplification tests, such as polymerase chain reaction for toxin B. Although more expensive than enzyme immunoassay testing, they are more accurate and early diagnosis and therapy will ultimately make them more cost effective.

Therapy

If possible, initial antibiotics should be discontinued. Recommended initial therapy for mild to moderate CDI is metronidazole, 500 mg three times a day for 10 days, unless there is a contraindication or intolerance to metronidazole. Patients should improve within 3 to 5 days, and be asymptomatic at the end of the treatment course.

Patients with severe CDI should receive initial therapy with oral vancomycin, 125 mg four times a day for 10 days. If there is no improvement in 3 to 5 days, the dose can be increased to 250 mg four times a day. Patients with severe and complicated CDI should be treated with high-dose oral vancomycin (500 mg four times a day) and intravenous metronidazole every 6 hours. Vancomycin enemas can be added in patients with an ileus. These patients are critically ill and should be managed in conjunction with a surgical team because some may need colectomy or diverting loop ileostomy if they do not respond to maximal medical therapy (**Fig. 3**).

Recurrent CDI

RCDI is CDI that recurs after treatment, usually within 30 days. Repeat antibiotics are needed to treat it. The first recurrence can be treated with the same antibiotic or an alternate, i.e. metronidazole or vancomycin. The second recurrence should be treated with a vancomycin pulse regimens. A good regimen is vancomycin 125 mg four times a day for ten days, followed by a single dose of vancomycin 125 mg orally every 3 days for 10 doses.

Nonantibiotic therapies are emerging as highly viable treatment strategies for recurrent or severe refractory disease. Fecal microbiota transplant, which involves the transference of stool from an uninfected donor to the colon of and individual with CDI, is currently recommended as second-line therapy for recurrent CDI.[22] Systematic review has demonstrated disease resolution in about 90% of cases, and closer to 98% secondary cure rate.[66,67] A recent review evaluated fecal microbiota transplant for recurrent CDI in a cohort of elderly patients older than age 65.[68] They found similar overall results, safety profile, and cure rates near 90%. There was no significant difference in cure rate between older and younger patients, and microbiologic studies correlated clinical remission with shift in fecal microbiota to resemble that of the donors.

Immunoglobulins targeted against toxins A and B have been evaluated as therapeutic options given the protective effect associated with innate humoral responses to *C difficile*. A phase 2 trial involving 200 patients showed CDI recurrence was lower among patients treated with monoclonal antibodies (7% compared with 25%), but did not alter the severity of disease.[69] Monoclonal antibodies remain unavailable, however, outside research settings.

PROPHYLAXIS

Effective prophylaxis against CDI remains elusive. Evidence is limited regarding probiotic formulations for prevention of incident or recurrent CDI. The most recent Cochrane

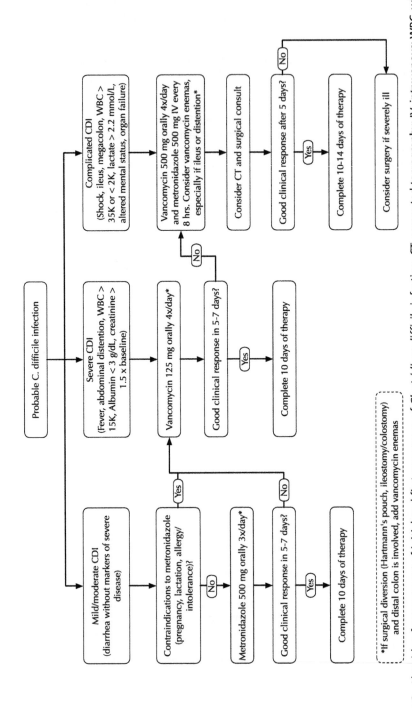

Fig. 3. Algorithm for treatment of initial and first recurrence of *Clostridium difficile* infection. CT, computed tomography; IV, intravenous; WBC, white blood cell. (*From* Knight CL, Surawicz CM. *Clostridium difficile* infection. Med Clin North Am 2013;97:530; with permission.)

Review analyzing 23 randomized trials investigating probiotics showed a 64% reduced risk of *C difficile*–associated diarrhea, although no difference in the rate of CDI.[70] Adverse events were reduced by 20% in the probiotic arm, and no safety issues were encountered. The data were strong enough to confer a moderate-strength recommendation for using probiotics as adjuncts to antibiotic therapy for short-term use in healthy and nonimmunocompromised patients. A recent large randomized controlled trial in the United Kingdom evaluated probiotic administration to elderly patients admitted to the hospital as prophylaxis against antibiotic-associated diarrhea or *C difficile*–associated diarrhea.[71] There was a statistically insignificant trend toward reduced *C difficile* diarrhea, but no evidence that probiotics prevented antibiotic-associated diarrhea. Thus, probiotics may serve an ancillary role to antibiotics in prevention of CDI; however, there is no evidence they provide effective prophylaxis. In addition, discretion must be used with careful analysis of the risks and benefits before therapeutic use of live organisms, especially in older patient populations. There are several reported cases of invasive *Lactobacillus* infections in elderly patients that are otherwise immunocompetent.[72,73] The most recent American College of Gastroenterology guidelines do not recommend adjunctive probiotic use, awaiting further conclusive data.

Several vaccines directed against *C difficile* toxins are currently under investigation. Vaccine administration to healthy volunteers results in antitoxin IgG elevated to levels associated with protection.[74] Vaccination strategies may prove problematic in older patients under typical protocols, however, because vaccine efficacy tends to decrease significantly after age 65 due to altered immune function.[75] A recent phase I study of an adjuvanted *C difficile* toxoid vaccine included a cohort of healthy elderly volunteers older than age 65.[76] Seroconversion was delayed in elderly compared with younger volunteers, and immunity subsequently declined more markedly in the elderly. Further studies are needed to determine the clinical significance, if any, of the age-related variance in vaccine response.

Treatment of asymptomatic carriers to prevent horizontal transmission is not recommended. Eradication of *C difficile* carriage is poor with metronidazole, and recolonization rates are high with vancomycin.[77] Treating carriers may in fact facilitate shedding of spores.[78]

PREVENTION

Infection control regimens and containment of contaminated environments are critical factors limiting transmission of *C difficile*. Although the vegetative form of the bacteria can survive minutes to hours depending on moisture levels, spores are highly resistant to routine sanitation methods[79] and can persist for up to 5 months.[80] Bleach solutions for surface decontamination effectively reduce *C difficile* spore concentrations and clinically reduce the rate of CDI.[40] Hand-hygiene with soap and water is imperative, because no antiseptic hand-wash or hand-rub agents are reliably sporicidal.[81] Contact precautions should be implemented until the time of discharge, because *C difficile* spores persist after resolution of diarrhea with shedding up to 6 weeks after therapy.[82]

Facility-wide policies to isolate patients with CDI to private rooms have been associated with lower organism prevalence.[83] Isolation may prove difficult in hospitals and long-term care facilities with limited availability of such rooms, but becomes especially important in preventing disease outbreak. Epidemiologic studies suggest that although incidence of CDI was lower in nursing homes than hospitals, the total number of cases was higher at nursing homes,[48] where CDI can be especially burdensome. According to the 2004 National Nursing Home Survey, 47.7% of residents were not continent of bowel and only 15.9% were fully independent in toileting.[84] CDI can lead to incontinence from the severity of diarrhea and the fecal urgency and frequency of toileting needs. The result is decreased quality of life, increased demand on nursing home personnel, and adverse consequences including susceptibility to pressure ulcers and falls.[85]

Reducing unnecessary antibiotic exposure is also an important intervention to prevent CDI, which are prescribed at higher rates in elderly patients with more acute and chronic diseases. Rates of inappropriate antibiotic use have been as high as 25% to 75% in long-term care facilities when assessing indication and duration of treatment.[86] Antibiotic stewardship programs that limit antimicrobial use have led to decreased rates of CDI in long-term care facilities[87] and the inpatient setting.[88–90]

SUMMARY

CDI remains a significant but preventable disease disproportionately affecting geriatric populations in the health care and community settings. Infections from C difficile are overcoming other health care–acquired infections, including methicillin-resistant S aureus and vancomycin-resistant Enterococcus. Elderly patients endure the overwhelming burden of morbidity and mortality from C difficile through mechanisms that are incompletely understood but likely multifactorial related to more comorbid diagnoses, increased pharmaceutical exposure, altered intestinal microbiota, and increased contact with health care environments. Early diagnosis, appropriate treatment, and ultimately prevention through infection control practices and optimization of therapeutic interventions are critical to minimizing the impact of disease for a rapidly aging population.

REFERENCES

1. Bartlett JG. Clinical practice. Antibiotic-associated diarrhea. N Engl J Med 2002; 346:334–9.
2. Thielman NM, Guerrant RL. Clinical practice. Acute infectious diarrhea. N Engl J Med 2004;350:38–47.
3. Miller BA, Chen LF, Sexton DJ, et al. Comparison of the burdens of hospital-onset, healthcare facility-associated Clostridium difficile infection and of healthcare-associated infection due to methicillin-resistant Staphylococcus aureus in community hospitals. Infect Control Hosp Epidemiol 2011;32:387–90.
4. Laffan AM, Bellantoni MF, Greenough WB, et al. Burden of Clostridium difficile-associated diarrhea in a long-term care facility. J Am Geriatr Soc 2006;54: 1068–73.
5. Bartlett JG. Antibiotic-associated diarrhea. Clin Infect Dis 1992;15:573–81.
6. Lucado J, Gould C, Elixhauser A. Clostridium difficile infections (CDI) in hospital stays. Healthcare Cost and Utilization Project, Agency for Healthcare Research and Quality Statistical Brief #124 2009.
7. McGlone SM, Bailey RR, Zimmer SM, et al. The economic burden of Clostridium difficile. Clin Microbiol Infect 2012;18:282–9.
8. Loo VG, Poirier L, Miller MA, et al. A predominantly clonal multi-institutional outbreak of Clostridium difficile-associated diarrhea with high morbidity and mortality. N Engl J Med 2005;353:2442–9.
9. McDonald LC, Killgore GE, Thompson A, et al. An epidemic, toxin gene-variant strain of Clostridium difficile. N Engl J Med 2005;353:2433–41.
10. Clements AC, Magalhães RJ, Tatem AJ, et al. Clostridium difficile PCR ribotype 027: assessing the risks of further worldwide spread. Lancet Infect Dis 2010;10: 395–404.

11. Gerding DN. *Clostridium difficile* 30 years on: what has, or has not, changed and why? Int J Antimicrob Agents 2009;33(Suppl 1):S2–8.

12. Miniño AM, Murphy SL, Xu J, et al. Deaths: final data for 2008. Natl Vital Stat Rep 2011;59:1–126.

13. Kyne L, Hamel MB, Polavaram R, et al. Health care costs and mortality associated with nosocomial diarrhea due to *Clostridium difficile*. Clin Infect Dis 2002; 34:346–53.

14. Kelly CP, Pothoulakis C, LaMont JT. *Clostridium difficile* colitis. N Engl J Med 1994;330:257–62.

15. Bartlett JG, Chang TW, Gurwith M, et al. Antibiotic-associated pseudomembranous colitis due to toxin-producing clostridia. N Engl J Med 1978;298:531–4.

16. Manges AR, Labbe A, Loo VG, et al. Comparative metagenomic study of alterations to the intestinal microbiota and risk of nosocomial *Clostridum difficile*-associated disease. J Infect Dis 2010;202:1877–84.

17. Thelestam M, Chaves-Olarte E. Cytotoxic effects of the *Clostridium difficile* toxins. Curr Top Microbiol Immunol 2000;250:85–96.

18. McFarland LV, Mulligan ME, Kwok RY, et al. Nosocomial acquisition of *Clostridium difficile* infection. N Engl J Med 1989;320:204–10.

19. Kyne L, Warny M, Qamar A, et al. Association between antibody response to toxin A and protection against recurrent *Clostridium difficile* diarrhoea. Lancet 2001;357:189–93.

20. Kyne L, Warny M, Qamar A, et al. Asymptomatic carriage of *Clostridium difficile* and serum levels of IgG antibody against toxin A. N Engl J Med 2000;342: 390–7.

21. Frasca D, Diaz A, Romero M, et al. Age effects on B cells and humoral immunity in humans. Ageing Res Rev 2011;10:330–5.

22. Surawicz CM, Brandt LJ, Binion DG, et al. Guidelines for diagnosis, treatment, and prevention of *Clostridium difficile* infections. Am J Gastroenterol 2013; 108:478–98 [quiz: 499].

23. Kim JH, Muder RR. *Clostridium difficile* enteritis: a review and pooled analysis of the cases. Anaerobe 2011;17:52–5.

24. McDonald LC, Owings M, Jernigan DB. *Clostridium difficile* infection in patients discharged from US short-stay hospitals, 1996-2003. Emerg Infect Dis 2006;12: 409–15.

25. Loo VG, Bourgault AM, Poirier L, et al. Host and pathogen factors for *Clostridium difficile* infection and colonization. N Engl J Med 2011;365:1693–703.

26. Hopkins MJ, Macfarlane GT. Changes in predominant bacterial populations in human faeces with age and with *Clostridium difficile* infection. J Med Microbiol 2002;51:448–54.

27. Rea MC, O'Sullivan O, Shanahan F, et al. *Clostridium difficile* carriage in elderly subjects and associated changes in the intestinal microbiota. J Clin Microbiol 2012;50:867–75.

28. Skraban J, Dzeroski S, Zenko B, et al. Gut microbiota patterns associated with colonization of different *Clostridium difficile* ribotypes. PLoS One 2013;8:e58005.

29. Hakim FT, Gress RE. Immunosenescence: deficits in adaptive immunity in the elderly. Tissue Antigens 2007;70:179–89.

30. Ginaldi L, Loreto MF, Corsi MP, et al. Immunosenescence and infectious diseases. Microbes Infect 2001;3:851–7.

31. Warny M, Vaerman JP, Avesani V, et al. Human antibody response to *Clostridium difficile* toxin A in relation to clinical course of infection. Infect Immun 1994;62: 384–9.

32. Solomon K, Martin AJ, O'Donoghue C, et al. Mortality in patients with *Clostridium difficile* infection correlates with host pro-inflammatory and humoral immune responses. J Med Microbiol 2013;62:1453–60.

33. Freeman J, Wilcox MH. Antibiotics and *Clostridium difficile*. Microbes Infect 1999;1:377–84.

34. Freeman J, Bauer MP, Baines SD, et al. The changing epidemiology of *Clostridium difficile* infections. Clin Microbiol Rev 2010;23:529–49.

35. Hensgens MP, Goorhuis A, Dekkers OM, et al. Time interval of increased risk for *Clostridium difficile* infection after exposure to antibiotics. J Antimicrob Chemother 2012;67:742–8.

36. Stevens V, Dumyati G, Fine LS, et al. Cumulative antibiotic exposures over time and the risk of *Clostridium difficile* infection. Clin Infect Dis 2011;53:42–8.

37. Srinivasan A, Fishman N. Antimicrobial stewardship 2012: science driving practice. Infect Control Hosp Epidemiol 2012;33:319–21.

38. Jacob JT, Gaynes RP. Emerging trends in antibiotic use in US hospitals: quality, quantification and stewardship. Expert Rev Anti Infect Ther 2010;8: 893–902.

39. Khanna S, Pardi DS, Aronson SL, et al. The epidemiology of community-acquired *Clostridium difficile* infection: a population-based study. Am J Gastroenterol 2012;107:89–95.

40. Weber DJ, Anderson DJ, Sexton DJ, et al. Role of the environment in the transmission of *Clostridium difficile* in health care facilities. Am J Infect Control 2013; 41:S105–10.

41. Salkind AR. *Clostridium difficile*: an update for the primary care clinician. South Med J 2010;103:896–902.

42. Bartlett JG. Historical perspectives on studies of *Clostridium difficile* and *C. difficile* infection. Clin Infect Dis 2008;46(Suppl 1):S4–11.

43. Riggs MM, Sethi AK, Zabarsky TF, et al. Asymptomatic carriers are a potential source for transmission of epidemic and nonepidemic *Clostridium difficile* strains among long-term care facility residents. Clin Infect Dis 2007;45:992–8.

44. Guerrero DM, Becker JC, Eckstein EC, et al. Asymptomatic carriage of toxigenic *Clostridium difficile* by hospitalized patients. J Hosp Infect 2013;85:155–8.

45. Yakob L, Riley TV, Paterson DL, et al. *Clostridium difficile* exposure as an insidious source of infection in healthcare settings: an epidemiological model. BMC Infect Dis 2013;13:376.

46. Shaughnessy MK, Micielli RL, DePestel DD, et al. Evaluation of hospital room assignment and acquisition of *Clostridium difficile* infection. Infect Control Hosp Epidemiol 2011;32:201–6.

47. Kim JH, Toy D, Muder RR. *Clostridium difficile* infection in a long-term care facility: hospital-associated illness compared with long-term care-associated illness. Infect Control Hosp Epidemiol 2011;32:656–60.

48. Campbell RJ, Giljahn L, Machesky K, et al. *Clostridium difficile* infection in Ohio hospitals and nursing homes during 2006. Infect Control Hosp Epidemiol 2009; 30:526–33.

49. Mylotte JM, Russell S, Sackett B, et al. Surveillance for *Clostridium difficile* infection in nursing homes. J Am Geriatr Soc 2013;61:122–5.

50. Berg AM, Kelly CP, Farraye FA. *Clostridium difficile* infection in the inflammatory bowel disease patient. Inflamm Bowel Dis 2013;19:194–204.

51. Neofytos D, Kobayashi K, Alonso CD, et al. Epidemiology, risk factors, and outcomes of *Clostridium difficile* infection in kidney transplant recipients. Transpl Infect Dis 2013;15:134–41.

52. Alonso CD, Dufresne SF, Hanna DB, et al. *Clostridium difficile* infection after adult autologous stem cell transplantation: a multicenter study of epidemiology and risk factors. Biol Blood Marrow Transplant 2013;19:1502–8.
53. O'Keefe SJ. Tube feeding, the microbiota, and *Clostridium difficile* infection. World J Gastroenterol 2010;16:139–42.
54. Bunchorntavakul C, Chavalitdhamrong D. Bacterial infections other than spontaneous bacterial peritonitis in cirrhosis. World J Hepatol 2012;4:158–68.
55. Eddi R, Malik MN, Shakov R, et al. Chronic kidney disease as a risk factor for *Clostridium difficile* infection. Nephrology (Carlton) 2010;15:471–5.
56. Southern WN, Rahmani R, Aroniadis O, et al. Postoperative *Clostridium difficile*-associated diarrhea. Surgery 2010;148:24–30.
57. Thorens J, Froehlich F, Schwizer W, et al. Bacterial overgrowth during treatment with omeprazole compared with cimetidine: a prospective randomised double blind study. Gut 1996;39:54–9.
58. Williams C. Occurrence and significance of gastric colonization during acid-inhibitory therapy. Best Pract Res Clin Gastroenterol 2001;15:511–21.
59. Kwok CS, Arthur AK, Anibueze CI, et al. Risk of *Clostridium difficile* infection with acid suppressing drugs and antibiotics: meta-analysis. Am J Gastroenterol 2012;107:1011–9.
60. Choudhry MN, Soran H, Ziglam HM. Overuse and inappropriate prescribing of proton pump inhibitors in patients with *Clostridium difficile*-associated disease. QJM 2008;101:445–8.
61. Dalton BR, Lye-Maccannell T, Henderson EA, et al. Proton pump inhibitors increase significantly the risk of *Clostridium difficile* infection in a low-endemicity, non-outbreak hospital setting. Aliment Pharmacol Ther 2009;29:626–34.
62. Rogers MA, Greene MT, Young VB, et al. Depression, antidepressant medications, and risk of *Clostridium difficile* infection. BMC Med 2013;11:121.
63. Naggie S, Miller BA, Zuzak KB, et al. A case-control study of community-associated *Clostridium difficile* infection: no role for proton pump inhibitors. Am J Med 2011;124:276.e1–7.
64. Motzkus-Feagans CA, Pakyz A, Polk R, et al. Statin use and the risk of *Clostridium difficile* in academic medical centres. Gut 2012;61:1538–42.
65. Cohen SH, Gerding DN, Johnson S, et al. Clinical practice guidelines for *Clostridium difficile* infection in adults: 2010 update by the Society for Healthcare Epidemiology of America (SHEA) and the Infectious Diseases Society of America (IDSA). Infect Control Hosp Epidemiol 2010;31:431–55.
66. Gough E, Shaikh H, Manges AR. Systematic review of intestinal microbiota transplantation (fecal bacteriotherapy) for recurrent *Clostridium difficile* infection. Clin Infect Dis 2011;53:994–1002.
67. Brandt LJ, Aroniadis OC, Mellow M, et al. Long-term follow-up of colonoscopic fecal microbiota transplant for recurrent *Clostridium difficile* infection. Am J Gastroenterol 2012;107:1079–87.
68. Burke KE, Lamont JT. Fecal transplantation for recurrent *Clostridium difficile* infection in older adults: a review. J Am Geriatr Soc 2013;61:1394–8.
69. Lowy I, Molrine DC, Leav BA, et al. Treatment with monoclonal antibodies against *Clostridium difficile* toxins. N Engl J Med 2010;362:197–205.
70. Goldenberg JZ, Ma SS, Saxton JD, et al. Probiotics for the prevention of *Clostridium difficile*-associated diarrhea in adults and children. Cochrane Database Syst Rev 2013;(5):CD006095.
71. Allen S, Wareham K, Wang D, et al. PWE-008 placide: probiotics in the prevention of antibiotic associated diarrhoea (AAD) and *Clostridium difficile* associated

diarrhoea (CDD) in elderly patients admitted to hospital: results of a large multi-centre RCT in the UK. Gut 2013;62:A133.

72. Salminen MK, Tynkkynen S, Rautelin H, et al. *Lactobacillus* bacteremia during a rapid increase in probiotic use of *Lactobacillus rhamnosus* GG in Finland. Clin Infect Dis 2002;35:1155–60.

73. Salminen MK, Rautelin H, Tynkkynen S, et al. *Lactobacillus* bacteremia, clinical significance, and patient outcome, with special focus on probiotic *L. rhamnosus* GG. Clin Infect Dis 2004;38:62–9.

74. Kotloff KL, Wasserman SS, Losonsky GA, et al. Safety and immunogenicity of increasing doses of a *Clostridium difficile* toxoid vaccine administered to healthy adults. Infect Immun 2001;69:988–95.

75. Dorrington MG, Bowdish DM. Immunosenescence and novel vaccination strategies for the elderly. Front Immunol 2013;4:171.

76. Greenberg RN, Marbury TC, Foglia G, et al. Phase I dose finding studies of an adjuvanted *Clostridium difficile* toxoid vaccine. Vaccine 2012;30:2245–9.

77. Johnson S, Homann SR, Bettin KM, et al. Treatment of asymptomatic *Clostridium difficile* carriers (fecal excretors) with vancomycin or metronidazole. A randomized, placebo-controlled trial. Ann Intern Med 1992;117:297–302.

78. Chang HT, Krezolek D, Johnson S, et al. Onset of symptoms and time to diagnosis of *Clostridium difficile*-associated disease following discharge from an acute care hospital. Infect Control Hosp Epidemiol 2007;28:926–31.

79. Russell AD. Bacterial spores and chemical sporicidal agents. Clin Microbiol Rev 1990;3:99–119.

80. Kim KH, Fekety R, Batts DH, et al. Isolation of *Clostridium difficile* from the environment and contacts of patients with antibiotic-associated colitis. J Infect Dis 1981;143:42–50.

81. Boyce JM, Pittet D. Guideline for hand hygiene in health-care settings. Recommendations of the Healthcare Infection Control Practices Advisory Committee and the HICPAC/SHEA/APIC/IDSA Hand Hygiene Task Force. Society for Healthcare Epidemiology of America/Association for Professionals in Infection Control/Infectious Diseases Society of America. MMWR Recomm Rep 2002; 51:1–45 [quiz: CE1–4].

82. Sethi AK, Al-Nassir WN, Nerandzic MM, et al. Persistence of skin contamination and environmental shedding of *Clostridium difficile* during and after treatment of *C. difficile* infection. Infect Control Hosp Epidemiol 2010;31:21–7.

83. Simor AE, Williams V, McGeer A, et al. Prevalence of colonization and infection with methicillin-resistant *Staphylococcus aureus* and vancomycin-resistant *Enterococcus* and of *Clostridium difficile* infection in Canadian hospitals. Infect Control Hosp Epidemiol 2013;34:687–93.

84. Jones AL, Dwyer LL, Bercovitz AR, et al. The National Nursing Home Survey: 2004 overview. Vital Health Stat 13 2009;(167):1–155.

85. Dubberke ER, Olsen MA. Burden of *Clostridium difficile* on the healthcare system. Clin Infect Dis 2012;55(Suppl 2):S88–92.

86. Nicolle LE, Bentley DW, Garibaldi R, et al. Antimicrobial use in long-term-care facilities. SHEA Long-Term-Care Committee. Infect Control Hosp Epidemiol 2000;21:537–45.

87. Jump RL, Olds DM, Seifi N, et al. Effective antimicrobial stewardship in a long-term care facility through an infectious disease consultation service: keeping a LID on antibiotic use. Infect Control Hosp Epidemiol 2012;33:1185–92.

88. Davey P, Brown E, Fenelon L, et al. Systematic review of antimicrobial drug prescribing in hospitals. Emerg Infect Dis 2006;12:211–6.

89. Aldeyab MA, Kearney MP, Scott MG, et al. An evaluation of the impact of antibiotic stewardship on reducing the use of high-risk antibiotics and its effect on the incidence of *Clostridium difficile* infection in hospital settings. J Antimicrob Chemother 2012;67:2988–96.
90. Davey P, Brown E, Fenelon L, et al. Interventions to improve antibiotic prescribing practices for hospital inpatients. Cochrane Database Syst Rev 2005;(4):CD003543.

Anorectal Physiology and Pathophysiology in the Elderly

Siegfried W.B. Yu, MD, Satish S.C. Rao, MD, PhD, FRCP (LON)*

KEYWORDS

- Anorectal pathophysiology • Elderly • Age-related cellular dysfunction
- Fecal incontinence • Constipation

KEY POINTS

- The key mechanisms underlying age-related cellular dysfunction include oxidative damage affecting the nucleotide pool and biochemical pathways associated with cell structure and function, and epigenetic alterations in gene expression that affect the plasticity of senescent cells.
- In the colons of human patients, age-related neuronal loss is also associated with an increased proportion of abnormal-appearing myenteric ganglia with cavities, which may contribute to disturbed colonic motility with aging.
- Aging is associated with a variety of effects on anorectal function. Healthy elderly women have demonstrated thinning of the internal anal sphincter, resulting in decreased resting and maximum squeeze pressure in the anal canal. Thickening of the external sphincter is also observed, but does not correlate with increased continence. In the absence of disease, age-related changes in the sphincter function of aging males appears minimal.

INTRODUCTION

Anorectal disorders such as fecal incontinence (FI), chronic constipation, dyssynergic defecation, fecal impaction, and overflow FI are highly prevalent in the elderly. These conditions significantly affect the quality of life, and pose a large health care burden. Estimates from the US Bureau of the Census indicate that the size of the United States population 85 years and older will increase from approximately 5 to 20 million between 2000 and 2050.[1] Although a benign condition, constipation can result in chronic illness with potentially serious complications (FI, impaction, and bowel perforation).[2] FI affects between 6% and 19% of elderly individuals aged 65 years and older living in

Grant Support: S.S.C. Rao is supported by a grant from National Institutes of Health, grant RO1 DK 57100-05NIHRO-1.

Division of Gastroenterology and Hepatology, Medical College of Georgia, Georgia Regents University, 1120 15th Street, Augusta, GA 30912, USA

* Corresponding author. Section of Gastroenterology and Hepatology, Medical College of Georgia, Georgia Regents University, BBR2540, 1120 15th Street, Augusta, GA 30912.
E-mail address: srao@gru.edu

the community and, unlike in younger patients, men and women are equally affected.[3] It is associated with significant social stigma and psychological distress; leads to dependency, poor health, and a high caregiver burden; and is a leading reason for nursing home placement for the elderly.[4] Although there is improved understanding of the mechanisms of some of these disorders, there is a significant lack of knowledge regarding normal and abnormal changes of anorectal function and the biological changes associated with aging. This article addresses the relevant structural and functional changes of the anorectum in the elderly, and discusses their implications for the pathogenesis of common anorectal disorders.

FUNCTIONAL ANATOMY AND PHYSIOLOGY

The colon has a well-established circadian rhythm, with a significant increase in motility after meals and after waking. During waking hours, the transverse/descending colon exhibits more activity, attributed to its role of mixing, storage, and salvaging digestive residue, while nocturnal activity is predominated by periodic rectal motor activity, which presumably acts as an intrinsic nocturnal brake that helps to maintain continence during sleep (**Fig. 1**).[5,6] Between 3 and 10 times a day, intermittent high-amplitude (>100 mm Hg) prolonged-duration propagating contractions (HAPCs) sweep through the colon, delivering fecal material into the rectum. The numbers of HAPCs are significantly decreased or absent in patients with slow-transit constipation, but whether these characteristics are different in the elderly is not known.[6]

The rectum acts as a reservoir for stool and as a pump for emptying stool, and has 3 involutions known as the valves of Houston. The lateral angulations of the sigmoid colon and valves of Houston provide a mechanical barrier that helps retard progression of stool, with the weight of the stool enhancing this barrier effect.[7] Stool volume and consistency are important, because patients with a weakened continence mechanism may be continent for firm stool but incontinent for liquid feces. Both the adaptive compliance of the rectum and rectal capacity are important for its reservoir function.[8]

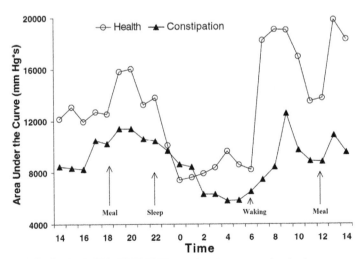

Fig. 1. A 24-hour profile of the mean area under the curve of colonic pressure waves in healthy and constipated patients. There is a significant increase in colonic motility after meals and after waking. (*From* Rao SS, Sadeghi P, Beaty J, et al. Ambulatory 24-hour colonic manometry in slow-transit constipation. Am J Gastroenterol 2004;99(12):2409; with permission.)

The anus is a muscular tube 2 to 4 cm in length, the upper anal canal being lined with mostly columnar epithelium, the same tissue that lines the rectum. About 1 cm above the dentate line there is a change from columnar to squamous epithelium in an area of 1 to 1.5 cm, called the transitional zone. The anal sphincter consists of the internal anal sphincter, a 0.3- to 0.5-cm thick expansion of the circular smooth muscle layer of the rectum, which is under involuntary control, and the external anal sphincter, a 0.6- to 1-cm thick expansion of the striated levator ani muscles, which is under voluntary control. The anus forms an angle with the axis of the rectum, approximately 90° at rest. With voluntary squeeze it becomes more acute, around 70°, and during defecation becomes more obtuse, at 110° to 130° (**Fig. 2**).[9]

The anus is normally closed by the tonic activity of the internal anal sphincter, which keeps the canal in the collapsed position to maintain continence.[10] When the rectal ampulla fills and induces distention, the sensory stimulus for evacuation releases the state of tonic contraction and begins the process of defecation. If volume increases rapidly over a short period, the accommodation response fails and leads to urgent emptying.[8]

The pelvic floor consists of the pubococcygeus, iliococcygeus, and puborectalis, a group of muscles that forms the levator ani. The pubococcygeus and iliococcygeus participate in continence by applying lateral pressure to narrow the levator hiatus. Recent work has shown that the puborectalis plays an integral role in maintaining continence, and is either scarred or damaged in women with FI.[11] The external anal sphincter is composed of multiple interrelated skeletal muscle loops that lie in close approximation to the levator ani and the muscles of the pelvic floor, and is under

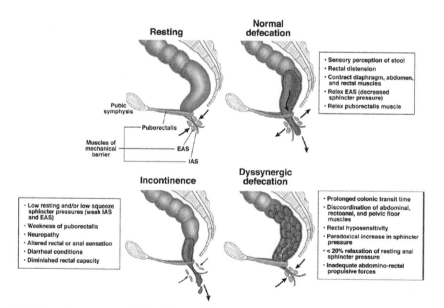

Fig. 2. Normal anatomy and physiology of the pelvic floor in the sagittal plane at rest, during defecation, and the key pathophysiologic changes in subjects with fecal incontinence and dyssynergic defecation. This profile shows the arrangement of the 3 anal muscles during rest and normal defecation, and the impairment that occurs with fecal incontinence and dyssynergic defecation. EAS, external anal sphincter; IAS, internal anal sphincter. (*From* Rao SS. Advances in diagnostic assessment of fecal incontinence and dyssynergic defecation. Clin Gastroenterol Hepatol 2010;8(11):911; with permission.)

voluntary control. This sphincter system contains 3 muscular loops that surround the anal canal. The external anal sphincter is innervated by the inferior hemorrhoidal branch of the pudendal nerve. Continuous tonic activity of the external anal sphincter and pelvic floor muscles has been recorded at rest and during sleep, which helps maintain fecal continence.[12]

The internal anal sphincter has both sympathetic and parasympathetic innervation. The parasympathetic nerves are inhibitory to the internal anal sphincter while the sympathetic outflow mediates contraction and relaxation.[13,14] Activity of the sphincters is the most important factor in maintaining anal continence. The internal anal sphincter is estimated to account for 52% to 85% of the pressure recorded in the high-pressure zone of the anal canal.[15] The hemorrhoidal cushions also play a significant physiologic role in protecting the anus, augmenting closure of the anal canal in response to increased abdominal pressure by engorging with increased inferior vena cava pressure, and contributes 15% to 20% of resting anal canal pressure, another important mechanism that preserves fecal continence.[16]

Three anal reflexes have been described: the rectoanal inhibitory reflex (RAIR), the rectoanal contractile reflex (RACR), and the sensorimotor response (SMR) (**Fig. 3**). These reflexes are probably mediated by the pudendal nerve and are subserved by the sacral spinal cord segments S1 to S4. The RAIR is characterized by differential anal relaxation along the anterior-posterior axis, longitudinally along the length of anal canal, and is dependent on the rectal distention volume. Multidimensional analyses demonstrate that there is specific asymmetry in the RAIR. Recent work shows that it is maximally seen at the internal anal sphincter pressure zone, and is characterized manometrically by the loss of anal canal pressure during rectal balloon distention (relaxation pressure), and the lowest anal canal pressure point of the reflex (residual pressure).[17] The SMR is a transient anal contraction primarily induced by the

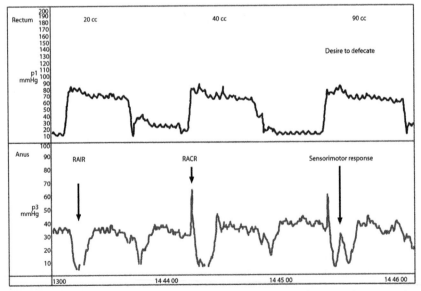

Fig. 3. Manometric representation of the rectoanal inhibitory reflex (RAIR), rectoanal contractile reflex (RACR), and sensorimotor response. (*From* Remes-Troche JM, De-Ocampo S, Valestin J, et al, Rectoanal reflexes and sensorimotor response in rectal hyposensitivity. Dis Colon Rectum 2010;53(7):1049; with permission.)

activation and contraction of the puborectalis muscle in response to the sensation of a desire to defecate.[18] It usually overlies the initial relaxation phase of the RAIR, and normally coincides with the onset of a sensation to defecate.[19] The RACR is a primordial reflex that prevents accidental release of rectal contents, and is mediated by the pelvic splanchnic and pudendal nerves.[20]

The sympathetic fibers to the rectum are derived from spinal cord segments L1 to L3. Parasympathetic fibers, which transmit the pathway for the sensation of rectal distention via the nervi erigentes, are derived from the spinal cord segments S2 to S4.[21] Rectal sensory perception is mediated by mechanoreceptors in the pelvic floor and wall itself.[22] Rectal hyposensitivity in patients with normal rectal compliance may reflect impaired afferent nerve function, whereas in patients with increased compliance it may be due to abnormal properties of the rectal wall.[22]

BIOPHYSIOLOGIC AND MOLECULAR EFFECTS OF AGING ON NEUROMUSCULAR FUNCTION

The key mechanisms underlying age-related cellular dysfunction include oxidative damage affecting the nucleotide pool and biochemical pathways associated with cell structure and function, and epigenetic alterations in gene expression that affect the plasticity of senescent cells. Endogenous reactive oxygen species are a mechanism of age-associated loss of myenteric neurons. The insufficient ability of cells to degrade damaged cytosolic macromolecules and organelles through autophagy results in accumulation of dysfunctional mitochondria in aged individuals that may result in cell death independent of the classic apoptosis pathway. The manipulation of factors that enhance autophagy function, such as SIRT1 and mTOR, has demonstrated significant increases in survival in several organisms, and emphasizes the role of autophagy in the regulation of life span.[23,24] In rodent models of aging, a significant reduction in the number of neurons occurs in the enteric nervous system, and is more prominent distally (60% in the colon and 40% in the small intestine).[25] In the *klotho* murine model of premature aging, fewer contractile proteins are expressed with generalized intestinal neuromuscular hypoplasia, in the presence of accelerated colonic and whole-gut transit, suggesting that decreased fecal output is due to reduced food intake rather than intestinal dysmotility.[26]

In the colons of human patients, age-related neuronal loss is also associated with an increased proportion of abnormal-appearing myenteric ganglia with cavities, which may contribute to disturbed colonic motility with aging.[27] Study of inhibitory innervation of human descending colon obtained at surgery has shown an age-related decrease in inhibitory junction potentials, suggesting a decrease in inhibitory nerves, neurotransmitter, and density of binding sites, and, alternatively, a possible change in the interaction of inhibitory neurotransmitters with the smooth muscle membrane.[28] Rectal sensory thresholds have been reported to be higher in aged healthy human volunteers, despite absence of changes in colorectal smooth muscle compliance and tone, and age is therefore suggested to be a potential confounding factor when studying rectal sensitivity.[29] It is possible that this observation may point to potential alterations in the normal accommodation reflexes involved in defecation.

The enteric nervous system (ENS) is complex, and enteric neurons are heterogeneous in their morphology, projections, and physiologic roles (**Table 1**).[30] In a study of the changes in innervation of the mouse internal anal sphincter with aging, Wang and colleagues[31] found a significant reduction in the density of neuronal nitric oxide synthetase (nNOS) and substance P (SP) immunoreactivity in the nerve fibers of aging murine internal anal sphincter circular muscle (3 vs 25 months), with significant

Table 1
Summary of the major types of myenteric and submucosal neurons in the mammalian gastrointestinal tract[a]

Main Functional Groups (% of Total, Guinea Pig[a])	Projections to Target Cells (Morphologic Classification)	Major Neurotransmitters and Modulators (Additional Neurochemical Markers)
Myenteric Plexus		
Intrinsic sensory neurons (26%)	Mucosal epithelium	Tachykinins/acetylcholine (calbindin)
Motor neurons that stimulate smooth muscle relaxation (18%)	Anal, to smooth muscle	Nitric oxide/vasoactive intestinal peptide/pituitary adenylate cyclase-activating polypeptide/adenosine triphosphate
Motor neurons that stimulate smooth muscle contraction (37%)	Oral, to smooth muscle	Acetylcholine/tachykinins
Interneurons (various types) (16%)	Oral and anal to other neurons	Acetylcholine/tachykinins/serotonin/neuropeptide Y/somatostatin
Neurons that project out of the gut (<1%)	Other autonomic ganglia	Acetylcholine
Submucosal Plexus		
Secretomotor/vasodilator neurons (noncholinergic) (45%)	Mucosal epithelium and intestinal blood vessels	Vasoactive intestinal peptide
Secretomotor/vasodilator neurons (44%)	Mucosal epithelium and blood vessels	Acetylcholine
Intrinsic sensory neurons (11%)	Myenteric and submucosal neurons, and epithelium	Thought to be tachykinin (express calbindin)

[a] Broadly similar proportions of the main neuronal types have been found in all species studied to date.

Adapted from Saffrey MJ. Ageing of the enteric nervous system. Mech Ageing Dev 2004;125(12):900.

decreases in the density of nNOS, vasoactive intestinal peptide (VIP), and SP in anal mucosal nerve fibers. These changes point to pathophysiologic alterations of anorectal motility and the defecation reflex with the aging process.

The submucosal plexus, which plays an important role in secretion and motility, has also been found to be impaired with age.[32] Phillips and colleagues[33] showed age-related increases in α-synuclein expression in the submucosal plexus, as well as significant decreases of glial cells, in Fischer 344 rats; this occurred in every region of the small and large intestine except for the rectum, which showed a nonsignificant decrease. The reason for the preferential sparing of the rectum is unclear. An interdependence between loss of glial cells and myenteric neuronal cell death was also found.[34] With age, the number and volume of interstitial cells of Cajal also decline, which reduces propulsive activity and sensorimotor functions within the gastrointestinal tract.[35]

Physiologic properties of isolated rat colonic smooth muscle cells demonstrate decreased average total Ca^{2+} current density with aging.[36] The decreased contractile properties of gastrointestinal smooth muscle with aging may be mediated by altered signal transduction pathways. Studies in aged rat colonic smooth muscle show that signal transduction may be affected by decreases in caveolin-1, a caveolae-specific protein that helps permit rapid and efficient coordination of signal cascades, which leads to smooth muscle contraction of the colon.[23] Deletion of growth hormone or its receptors has been shown to extend longevity, and expression is associated with smooth muscle cell proliferation and collagen synthesis in intestinal smooth muscle in rat models of intestinal growth and colonic inflammation.[37] The distribution of elastin and collagen has also been found to be increased around the myenteric plexus in the aging human colon, and may affect the ability to accommodate gut contents.[38]

In summary, significant alterations in age-related enteric neuronal structure and function have been observed, which offer a potential explanation for some of the disorders seen in the elderly.

IMPLICATIONS OF AGING NEUROMUSCULAR FUNCTION ON ANORECTAL DISORDERS

Although gastrointestinal functions are generally well preserved with aging, the progressive neuronal loss, and extrinsic factors such as diet, immobility, comorbidity, and the effects of medication, as well as previous trauma such as obstetric sphincter injury or back injury, may predispose the elderly to an impairment of colorectal sensorimotor function. In addition, the clinical impact of comorbid conditions has a significant effect on gastrointestinal muscular function, although these effects are heterogeneous and not clearly defined (**Table 2**).[39]

Aging is associated with a variety of effects on anorectal function. Healthy elderly women have demonstrated thinning of the internal anal sphincter, resulting in decreased resting and maximum squeeze pressure in the anal canal. Thickening of the external sphincter is also observed, but does not correlate with increased continence. In the absence of disease, age-related changes in the sphincter function of aging males appears minimal.[40,41] Increasing age is also associated with a more positive

Table 2 Physiologic changes in the elderly			
Structure	**Proposed Change**	**Pathophysiologic Significance**	**Clinical Problem**
Number of HAPCs	Decreased	Decreased colonic propulsion	Constipation
Colonic transit time	Prolonged	Slow colon transit	Constipation
Internal anal sphincter	Thinning/atrophy	Weak sphincter	Fecal seepage/incontinence
External anal sphincter	Thinning/atrophy	Weak sphincter	Urgency/incontinence
Pudendal nerve function	Decreased	Impairment of colorectal sensorimotor function	Fecal seepage/incontinence
Rectal sensation	Decreased	Impairment of colorectal sensorimotor function	Fecal seepage/incontinence
Rectal compliance	Decreased	Impaired reservoir function	Urgency/incontinence
Anal sphincter length	Decreased	Weak sphincter	Fecal seepage/urgency/incontinence
Rectal capacity	Decreased	Impaired reservoir function	Urgency/incontinence

Abbreviation: HAPCs, high-amplitude (>100 mm Hg) prolonged-duration propagating contractions.

rectoanal gradient during simulated evacuation and a shorter balloon expulsion time in asymptomatic women.[42] There is an increase in collagen in the colon wall that is accompanied by a decrease in tensile strength, which may predispose to mucosal herniation and decreased reservoir function.[8] Age-related reductions in basal and maximum anal sphincter tone, decreased compliance of the rectal vault, reduced rectal sensation, and increased perineal descent also occur.

CONSTIPATION AND DYSSYNERGIC DEFECATION

Slow colonic transit and increased frequency of segmenting contractions may result in increased water resorption and hard feces. Decreased fiber intake also predisposes to the production of hard feces and excessive straining. When traditional approaches, including a high-fiber diet and over-the-counter laxatives, have not helped, and obstruction, secondary to conditions such as colon cancer, has been excluded, an assessment of colonic transit time (CTT) with radiopaque markers (ROMs) and/or anorectal manometry should be performed. Although widely available, the utility of ROMs in assessing CTT for slow-transit constipation (STC) in the elderly is limited. Furthermore, there is significant overlap between STC and dyssynergia, with approximately 60% of patients with dyssynergic defecation showing delayed CTT. A newer technology, the wireless motility capsule (WMC), which measures pH, temperature, and pressure, has emerged as a useful test in the evaluation of STC. It has better sensitivity in comparison with ROMs (86% vs 28%), and good specificity (89%). A recent study using this modality showed that older constipated patients had slower transit than older healthy controls.[43]

FECAL INCONTINENCE

In the American College of Gastroenterology (ACG) Practice Guidelines, Rao[10] proposed 3 clinical subtypes of FI (**Table 3**). There is overlap between these 3 groups, but making a clinical distinction could help in assessing the underlying etiology and guiding investigation and management.

FI is defined as the involuntary passage of fecal matter through the anus, or the inability to control this discharge. In elderly hospitalized patients, contributing factors to FI include fecal loading (57%), functional disability (83%), loose stools (67%), and cognitive impairment (43%). The distribution of factors appears to differ in the nursing home setting, where cognitive impairment is significantly more common (up to 87%).[44] Contributing factors in both inpatients and outpatients include traumatic anal injury,

Table 3 Subtypes of fecal incontinence		
Type	Clinical Description	Potential Mechanism(s)
Passive incontinence	The involuntary discharge of stool or gas without awareness	Weak IAS and EAS Neuropathy Rectal hyposensitivity
Urge incontinence	The discharge of fecal matter despite active attempts to retain bowel contents	Weak IAS and EAS Rectal hypersensitivity Impaired rectal compliance
Fecal seepage	The leakage of stool following otherwise normal evacuation	Dyssynergia Rectal hyposensitivity Neuropathy

Abbreviations: EAS, external anal sphincter; IAS, internal anal sphincter.

neurologic deficits, inflammatory conditions, and defecatory disturbances associated with constipation and diarrhea. There is an important connection between FI and urinary incontinence (UI), or dual incontinence, and the strongest association is age older than 80 years, followed by depression, neurologic disease, functional limitation, multiparity, and heavier fetal birth weight.[45] One study found that in women who had suffered a third-degree or fourth-degree obstetric tear, 21% were incontinent at a mean of 18 months' follow-up.[46] A survey-based study reported that at long-term follow-up in women who had suffered a third-degree obstetric tear (at least 10 years), 53% of respondents complained of fecal incontinence.[47] UI is also an independent risk factor for developing FI in both community-dwelling and institutionalized adults.[48,49] Retrospective and survey data suggest that sacral nerve neuromodulation can improve dual incontinence (FI and UI), suggesting a common etiology.[50,51]

Constipation plays an integral role in the development of FI, which can result from fecal impaction and subsequent overflow FI, incompetence of internal anal sphincter, decreased rectal or anal sensation, and other structural pelvic floor or anorectal neuromuscular dysfunction caused by prior trauma from surgery or irradiation.[41] Loss of the endovascular cushions, impaired anorectal sensation, poor rectal compliance, compromised accommodation, or neuropathy affecting the pudendal, sacral, spinal, or central nervous system may also contribute to incontinence. Failure to perceive stool in the rectum may produce severe urgency to defecate or leakage of stool, especially when access to toileting is limited. Other problems common in the elderly that require further study include neuropathy, excessive perineal descent, rectocele, rectal mucosal intussusception, and prolapse.[52,53]

SUMMARY

There are exciting advances in our understanding of the physiology and cellular biology of aging and anorectal neuromuscular function. However, much work remains: this includes a better characterization of common disorders and their phenotypes, a better understanding of the clinical factors that contribute to the burden of anorectal disorders, and more knowledge of the underlying genetic, molecular, and biological changes that occur with aging. There is also an urgent need for further longitudinal physiologic, structural, and neurophysiologic studies in women following obstetric trauma and/or pregnancy, thus to better understand the impact of trauma on the aging process. Continued progress in this field, and a clear understanding of what is currently known, will pave the way for more accurate diagnosis and a rational approach to the treatment of these disorders.

REFERENCES

1. Campion EW. The oldest old. N Engl J Med 1994;330(25):1819–20.
2. Belsey J, Greenfield S, Candy D, et al. Systematic review: impact of constipation on quality of life in adults and children. Aliment Pharmacol Ther 2010;31(9): 938–49.
3. Goode PS, Burgio KL, Halli AD, et al. Prevalence and correlates of fecal incontinence in community-dwelling older adults. J Am Geriatr Soc 2005;53(4): 629–35.
4. Santos-Eggimann B, Cirilli NC, Monachon JJ. Frequency and determinants of urgent requests to home care agencies for community-dwelling elderly. Home Health Care Serv Q 2003;22(1):39–53.
5. Rao SS, Sadeghi P, Beaty J, et al. Ambulatory 24-h colonic manometry in healthy humans. Am J Physiol Gastrointest Liver Physiol 2001;280(4):G629–39.

6. Rao SS, Sadeghi P, Beaty J, et al. Ambulatory 24-hour colonic manometry in slow-transit constipation. Am J Gastroenterol 2004;99(12):2405–16.
7. Jorge JM, Habr-Gama A. Anatomy and Embryology. In: Beck DE, Roberts PL, Saclarides TJ, et al, editors. The ASCRS Textbook of Colon and Rectal Surgery. New York: Springer; 2011. p. 1–22.
8. Schouten W, Gordon PH. Physiology. In: Gordon PH, Nivatvongs S, editors. Principles and practice of surgery for the colon, rectum, and anus. New York, London: Informa healthcare; 2007. p. 29–61.
9. Rao SS. Advances in diagnostic assessment of fecal incontinence and dyssynergic defecation. Clin Gastroenterol Hepatol 2010;8(11):910–9.
10. Rao SS. Diagnosis and management of fecal incontinence. American College of Gastroenterology Practice Parameters Committee. Am J Gastroenterol 2004; 99(8):1585–604.
11. Chase S, Mittal R, Jesudason MR, et al. Anal sphincter repair for fecal incontinence: experience from a tertiary care centre. Indian J Gastroenterol 2010; 29(4):162–5.
12. Kumar D, Waldron D, Williams NS, et al. Prolonged anorectal manometry and external anal sphincter electromyography in ambulant human subjects. Dig Dis Sci 1990;35(5):641–8.
13. Gutierrez J, Shank AN. Autonomic control of the internal anal sphincter in man. Fifth International Symposium on Gastrointestinal Motility. Herentals (Belgium): Typoff Press; 1975.
14. Marcello P. Diseases of the Anorectum. In: Feldman M, Brandt LJ, editors. Sleisenger and Fordtran's gastrointestinal and liver disease. Philadelphia: Saunders Elsevier; 2010. p. 2257–74.
15. Ferrara A, Pemberton JH, Levin KE, et al. Relationship between anal canal tone and rectal motor activity. Dis Colon Rectum 1993;36(4):337–42.
16. Cintron J, Abacarian H. Benign anorectal: hemorrhoids. In: Wolff B, Fleshman JW, editors. The ASCRS of Colon and Rectal Surgery. New York: Springfer-Verlag; 2007. p. 156–77.
17. Cheeney G, Nguyen M, Valestin J, et al. Topographic and manometric characterization of the recto-anal inhibitory reflex. Neurogastroenterol Motil 2012;24(3): e147–54.
18. Cheeney G, Remes-Troche JM, Attaluri A, et al. Investigation of anal motor characteristics of the sensorimotor response (SMR) using 3-D anorectal pressure topography. Am J Physiol Gastrointest Liver Physiol 2011;300(2):G236–40.
19. De-Ocampo S, Remes-Troche JM, Miller MJ, et al. Rectoanal sensorimotor response in humans during rectal distension. Dis Colon Rectum 2007;50(10): 1639–46.
20. Remes-Troche JM, De-Ocampo S, Valestin J, et al. Rectoanal reflexes and sensorimotor response in rectal hyposensitivity. Dis Colon Rectum 2010;53(7): 1047–54.
21. Nivatvongs S, Gordon PH. Surgical anatomy. In: Gordon PH, Nivatvongs S, editors. Principles and practice of surgery for the colon, rectum, and anus. New York, London: Informa Healthcare; 2007. p. 1–27.
22. Gladman MA, Dvorkin LS, Lunniss PJ, et al. Rectal hyposensitivity: a disorder of the rectal wall or the afferent pathway? An assessment using the barostat. Am J Gastroenterol 2005;100(1):106–14.
23. Bitar K, Greenwood-Van Meerveld B, Saad R, et al. Aging and gastrointestinal neuromuscular function: insights from within and outside the gut. Neurogastroenterol Motil 2011;23(6):490–501.

24. Camilleri M, Cowen T, Koch TR. Enteric neurodegeneration in ageing. Neuro-gastroenterol Motil 2008;20(3):185–96.

25. Wade PR. Aging and neural control of the GI tract. I. Age-related changes in the enteric nervous system. Am J Physiol Gastrointest Liver Physiol 2002;283(3): G489–95.

26. Asuzu DT, Hayashi Y, Izbeki F, et al. Generalized neuromuscular hypoplasia, reduced smooth muscle myosin and altered gut motility in the klotho model of premature aging. Neurogastroenterol Motil 2011;23(7):e309–23.

27. Hanani M, Fellig Y, Udassin R, et al. Age-related changes in the morphology of the myenteric plexus of the human colon. Auton Neurosci 2004;113(1–2):71–8.

28. Koch TR, Carney JA, Go VL, et al. Inhibitory neuropeptides and intrinsic inhib-itory innervation of descending human colon. Dig Dis Sci 1991;36(6):712–8.

29. Lagier E, Delvaux M, Vellas B, et al. Influence of age on rectal tone and sensitivity to distension in healthy subjects. Neurogastroenterol Motil 1999;11(2):101–7.

30. Saffrey MJ. Ageing of the enteric nervous system. Mech Ageing Dev 2004; 125(12):899–906.

31. Wang C, Houghton MJ, Gamage PP, et al. Changes in the innervation of the mouse internal anal sphincter during aging. Neurogastroenterol Motil 2013; 25(7):e469–77.

32. Phillips RJ, Pairitz JC, Powley TL. Age-related neuronal loss in the submuco-sal plexus of the colon of Fischer 344 rats. Neurobiol Aging 2007;28(7): 1124–37.

33. Phillips RJ, Martin FN, Billingsley CN, et al. Alpha-synuclein expression patterns in the colonic submucosal plexus of the aging Fischer 344 rat: implications for biopsies in aging and neurodegenerative disorders? Neurogastroenterol Motil 2013;25(9):e621–33.

34. Phillips RJ, Kieffer EJ, Powley TL. Loss of glia and neurons in the myenteric plexus of the aged Fischer 344 rat. Anat Embryol (Berl) 2004;209(1):19–30.

35. Gomez-Pinilla PJ, Gibbons SJ, Sarr MG, et al. Changes in interstitial cells of Cajal with age in the human stomach and colon. Neurogastroenterol Motil 2011;23(1):36–44.

36. Xiong Z, Sperelakis N, Noffsinger A, et al. Changes in calcium channel current densities in rat colonic smooth muscle cells during development and aging. Am J Physiol 1993;265(3 Pt 1):C617–25.

37. Mahavadi S, Flynn RS, Grider JR, et al. Amelioration of excess collagen Ialphal, fibrosis, and smooth muscle growth in TNBS-induced colitis in IGF-I(+/-) mice. Inflamm Bowel Dis 2011;17(3):711–9.

38. Gomes OA, de Souza RR, Liberti EA. A preliminary investigation of the effects of aging on the nerve cell number in the myenteric ganglia of the human colon. Gerontology 1997;43(4):210–7.

39. Firth M, Prather CM. Gastrointestinal motility problems in the elderly patient. Gastroenterology 2002;122(6):1688–700.

40. Gundling F, Seidl H, Scalercio N, et al. Influence of gender and age on anorectal function: normal values from anorectal manometry in a large caucasian popula-tion. Digestion 2010;81(4):207–13.

41. Hall K. Effect of aging on gastrointestinal function. In: Halter JB, Tinetti ME, Studenski S, et al, editors. Hazzard's geriatric medicine and gerontology. New York: McGraw Hill; 2009. p. 1059–64.

42. Noelting J, Ratuapli SK, Bharucha AE, et al. Normal values for high-resolution anorectal manometry in healthy women: effects of age and significance of rec-toanal gradient. Am J Gastroenterol 2012;107(10):1530–6.

43. Rao SS, Coss-Adame E, Valestin J, et al. Evaluation of constipation in older adults: radioopaque markers (ROMs) versus wireless motility capsule (WMC). Arch Gerontol Geriatr 2012;55(2):289–94.

44. Akpan A, Gosney MA, Barret J. Factors contributing to fecal incontinence in older people and outcome of routine management in home, hospital and nursing home settings. Clin Interv Aging 2007;2(1):139–45.

45. Matthews CA, Whitehead WE, Townsend MK, et al. Risk factors for urinary, fecal, or dual incontinence in the nurses' health study. Obstet Gynecol 2013;122(3): 539–45.

46. Tjandra JJ, Chan MK, Kwok SY, et al. Predictive factors for faecal incontinence after third or fourth degree obstetric tears: a clinico-physiologic study. Colorectal Dis 2008;10(7):681–8.

47. Samarasekera DN, Bekhit MT, Wright Y, et al. Long-term anal continence and quality of life following postpartum anal sphincter injury. Colorectal Dis 2008; 10(8):793–9.

48. Halland M, Koloski NA, Jones M, et al. Prevalence correlates and impact of fecal incontinence among older women. Dis Colon Rectum 2013;56(9):1080–6.

49. Ditah I, Devaki P, Luma HN, et al. Prevalence, trends, and risk factors for fecal incontinence in US adults, 2005-2010. Clin Gastroenterol Hepatol 2013. pii: S1542-3565(13)01084-7. [Epub ahead of print].

50. Faucheron JL, Chodez M, Boillot B. Neuromodulation for fecal and urinary incontinence: functional results in 57 consecutive patients from a single institution. Dis Colon Rectum 2012;55(12):1278–83.

51. Caremel R, Damon H, Ruffion A, et al. Can sacral neuromodulation improve minor incontinence symptoms in doubly incontinent patients successfully treated for major incontinence symptoms? Urology 2012;79(1):80–5.

52. Leung FW, Schnelle J, Rao SC. Fecal incontinence. In: Capezuti EA, Siegler EL, Mezey MD, editors. Encyclopedia of elder care. New York: Springer Publishing Company; 2008. p. 303–5.

53. Leung FW, Rao SS. Approach to fecal incontinence and constipation in older hospitalized patients. Hosp Pract (1995) 2011;39(1):97–104.

Constipation
Understanding Mechanisms and Management

Vanessa C. Costilla, MD[a], Amy E. Foxx-Orenstein, DO[b],*

KEYWORDS

- Chronic constipation • Constipation testing • Anorectal manometry
- Dyssynergic defecation • Pelvic floor dysfunction • Outlet dysfunction
- Slow transit constipation

KEY POINTS

- Patients usually have a broader definition of constipation than physicians that encompasses myriad symptoms, including hard stools, feeling of incomplete evacuation, abdominal discomfort, bloating and distension, and excessive straining.
- There are 3 primary types of constipation: functional, slow transit, and outlet dysfunction, and many secondary causes.
- Diagnostic testing is not routinely recommended in the initial evaluation of constipation in the absence of alarm signs and should be targeted at symptoms or signs elicited in the history or physical that suggest an organic process.
- Because sedentary lifestyle and low-fiber diets are associated with constipation, self-management strategies of lifestyle changes that include increased exercise, high-fiber diets, and toilet training are often effective first-line management.
- Fiber and fiber supplements can worsen symptoms in some types of constipation.
- A variety of over-the-counter and prescription medications with unique mechanisms of action are available to remedy constipation.

INTRODUCTION

Constipation is one of the most common gastrointestinal disorders seen by gastroenterologists and primary care physicians. Symptoms of constipation occur frequently, with the greatest prevalence in the elderly. The prevalence in adults older than 60 years is 33%, whereas the overall prevalence among adults of all ages is about 16%.[1] Constipation is found more frequently in women[2] and in lower socioeconomic populations.

No funding.
No conflict of interest.
[a] Department of Internal Medicine, Mayo Clinic in Arizona, Scottsdale, AZ, USA; [b] Division of Gastroenterology, Mayo Clinic in Arizona, 13400 East Shea Boulevard, Scottsdale, AZ 85259, USA
* Corresponding author.
E-mail address: foxx-orenstein.amy@mayo.edu

Constipation reduces quality of life and poses a large economic burden, with more than \$820 million spent on laxatives each year.[3] Complications of constipation include hemorrhoids, fecal impaction, stercoral ulcers, fecal incontinence, rectal prolapse, volvulus, and excessive perineal or inadequate perineal descent. These complications often lead to emergency department visits and hospitalizations. The mechanisms and management of chronic constipation in the elderly are the focus of this article.

Chronic Constipation: Definitions

Physicians and patients often have different definitions of constipation. Physicians typically define chronic constipation as infrequent bowel movements, usually less than 3 per week, for at least 3 of the prior 12 months. Patients usually have a broader definition that encompasses myriad symptoms including hard stools, feeling of incomplete evacuation, abdominal discomfort, bloating and distension, excessive straining, sense of anorectal blockage during defecation, and the need for manual maneuvers.[1]

Primary Constipation

Chronic constipation can be divided into 2 main categories: primary and secondary. Primary constipation is further divided into 3 main types: functional, outlet dysfunction, and slow transit constipation. There can be overlap of primary types of constipation.

- Functional constipation is diagnosed using the Rome III criteria (**Box 1**). Functional idiopathic constipation is distinct from constipation-predominant irritable bowel syndrome (C-IBS) (**Box 2**), based on the severity of abdominal pain. C-IBS is characterized by abdominal pain or discomfort that improves with defecation.[4]
- Outlet dysfunction (also called *defecation disorders* and *pelvic floor dysfunction*) encompasses several defecation disorders in which the patient experiences difficult or unsatisfactory expulsion of stool from the rectum. Several causes exist, including presence of an anal fissure or stricture, hemorrhoids, rectocele, enterocele, impaired descent (excessive or inadequate), and dyssynergic defecation.[5] Dyssynergic defecation is the impaired relaxation and coordination of abdominal and pelvic floor muscles during evacuation.

Box 1
Functional constipation: Rome III criteria

1. Must include 2 or more of the following:
   a. Straining during at least 25% of defecations
   b. Lumpy or hard stools in at least 25% of defecations
   c. Sensation of incomplete evacuation for at least 25% of defecations
   d. Sensation of anorectal obstruction/blockage for at least 25% of defecations
   e. Manuel maneuvers to facilitate at least 25% of defecations (eg, digital evacuation, support of the pelvic floor)
   f. Fewer than 3 defecations per week
2. Loose stools are rarely present without the use of laxatives
3. Insufficient stools are rarely present without the use of laxatives
4. Criteria fulfilled for the last 3 months with symptom onset at least 6 months prior to diagnosis.[4]

Box 2
Irritable bowel syndrome: constipation predominant

Recurrent abdominal pain or discomfort (uncomfortable sensation not described as pain) at least 3 days per month in the last 3 months associated with 2 or more of the following:

1. Improvement with defecation

2. Onset associated with a change in frequency of stool

3. Onset associated with a change in form (appearance) of stool

4. Less than 25% of bowel movements were loose stools

5. Criterion fulfilled for at least 6 months prior to diagnosis.[4]

- Slow-transit constipation (also called *delayed transit* and *colonoparesis*) is defined as prolonged stool transit (>3 days) through the colon.[6] Patients typically have prolonged time between bowel movements, experience lack of urge to defecate, abdominal distension, and worse symptoms with a high-fiber diet.

Secondary Constipation

Secondary constipation may be caused by diet, medications, and underlying medical conditions (**Table 1**). Diets low in fiber and low fluid intake are associated with increased constipation. Elderly patients who often have a decreased appetite or

Table 1
Secondary causes of constipation

Medications	Neurologic and Myopathic Disorders	Other Conditions Associated with Constipation
Analgesics: *opiates, nonsteroidal anti-inflammatory agents*	Diabetes mellitus	Anorexia
Anticholinergic agents: antihistamines, belladonna	Parkinson's disease	Hypothyroidism
Anticonvulsants: carbamazepine	Connective tissue disorders	Pregnancy
Antihypertensives: calcium channel blockers (verapamil), diuretics, central acting agents (clonidine), β-blockers	Central nervous system lesions (stroke, spinal or gangilion tumor)	Psychological and psychiatric disorders
Antiparkinsonian agents: dopamine agents, benztropine	Amyloidosis	Paraneoplastic syndromes
Antispasmodics	Hirschprung's disease	Pseudo-obstruction
Antidepressants: tricyclic agents, monoamine oxidase inhibitors	Autoimmune	—
Antipsychotics	Chagas disease	—
Metal ion containing agents: antacids, sucralfate, ferrous sulfate	—	—

medical conditions that cause them to have poor intake, such as Alzheimer's dementia, are at especially high risk for dehydration that can lead to constipation.

Several medications are associated with constipation, including anticholinergic drugs, opioids, calcium-channel blockers, and nonsteroidal anti-inflammatory drugs. Anticholinergic drugs can decrease intestinal smooth-muscle contractility.[7] Calcium-channel blockers, especially verapamil, are notorious for causing severe constipation by causing rectosigmoid dysmotility.[8] Elderly patients are often on several of these medications simultaneously.

Several diseases are associated with constipation, including hypothyroidism, diabetes mellitus, and Parkinson's. Rare causes of constipation include amyloidosis and paraneoplastic syndromes. Paraneoplastic syndromes can cause pseudo-obstruction in some patients.

CLINICAL EVALUATION

Evaluation of constipation begins with a detailed history and physical examination, including a visual and digital anal examination. This initial assessment will help identify primary and secondary causes of constipation and the presence of alarm symptoms (**Box 3**). A thorough visual inspection can identify excoriation, hemorrhoids, anal asymmetry, and anal halo, a circumferential thickening of the anus that occurs with rectal prolapse. When bearing down as if to evacuate, one can assess the degree of perineal descent and the presence of rectal prolapse. The digital rectal examination allows for recognition of anatomic abnormalities. Sharp knifelike pain during the digital rectal examination indicates active mucosal injury, such as acute or chronic fissure, ulcer, or inflammation. Fecal impaction, often masked by loose stool or overflow (paradoxic) incontinence, can also be recognized with the digital rectal examination.

Diagnostic Testing

Diagnostic testing for constipation is not routinely recommended early on in the absence of alarm signs. Also, a person's age, functional status, ability to perform testing, and whether results will alter the treatment are considered. A treat-and-test approach is practical and cost effective when testing can be pursued in patients refractory to conservative treatment. Diagnostic testing is often targeted at symptoms or signs elicited in the history or physical that suggest an organic process and should be used if the information gained is apt to alter treatment. Not all patients require the same diagnostic approach.

When alarm symptoms are present, a dedicated evaluation of the colon with colonoscopy, or in selected cases, computed tomographic colography or flexible

---

Box 3
Alarm signs and symptoms

Involuntary weight loss

Hematochezia

Family history of colon cancer or inflammatory bowel disease

Positive fecal occult blood testing

Iron deficiency anemia

Change in symptoms

Nocturnal symptoms

sigmoidoscopy, should be performed. Colonoscopy is indicated in all patients older than 50 years who have never had colorectal cancer screening. Colorectal cancer screening should cease when patients have less than a 10-year life expectancy.

- Anorectal manometry systems quantify internal and external anal sphincter function at rest and during defecatory maneuvers, rectal sensation, and compliance.[9] Anorectal manometry, along with the rectal balloon expulsion test should be performed in patients who do not respond to laxatives or empiric medical therapy for constipation.[1] It may also aid in assessing an objective response to biofeedback therapy or neuromuscular training in patients with dyssynergic defecation. The balloon expulsion test can help identify outlet obstruction but does not exclude a functional or slow transit disorder.
- A colonic transit study objectively measures the speed of stool movement through the colon. Methods to measure colonic transit are radiopaque markers (Sitzmarks), colonic scintigraphy, and wireless motility capsule. These tests are useful for objectively confirming a patients' subjective complaint of constipation or decreased bowel frequency, confirming slow transit, and for documentation of regional delays in transit.[10] The wireless motility capsule or SmartPill is a data recording device that provides information on intestinal pH and transit times of the stomach, small bowel, and colon, which can help exclude a more global gastrointestinal transit disorder.[11]
- Standard defecography provides dynamic evaluation of the pelvic floor and can indicate the presence of failed evacuation caused by various outlet disorders including dyssynergia, rectal prolapse, enterocele, rectocele, cystocele, and degree of perineal descent. Dynamic pelvic magnetic resonance imaging is the only imaging modality that can evaluate global pelvic floor anatomy and the anal sphincter without radiation exposure.[12]
- Colonic manometry can be considered in adults with refractory constipation unresponsive to conventional treatment.[13] Colonic manometry, available mostly in tertiary care centers, may help identify colonic neuropathy, myopathy, or normal colonic function before consideration of colectomy in patients with severe constipation.

NONPHARMACOLOGIC MANAGEMENT OF CONSTIPATION

Because sedentary lifestyle and low-fiber diets are associated with constipation, self-management strategies of lifestyle changes that include increased exercise, high-fiber diets, and toilet training are often effective first-line management. Patients should be instructed to recognize and respond to the urge to defecate, especially in the morning. A regimented daily routine that ends with an evening fiber supplement and begins with mild physical activity, a hot caffeinated beverage, and high-fiber breakfast within an hour of arising takes advantage of known factors that stimulate intestinal motility and the gastrocolic reflex to facilitate defecation.[6]

Dietary Changes

The recommended dose of fiber intake per day is 25 to 30 g; most Americans consume less than half of this amount. Increased fiber consumption and hydration is the first line of therapy for patients with chronic constipation. Patients should strive to increase their dietary fiber by incorporating foods such as prunes, bananas, kiwis, other fruits, vegetables, grains, and bran. Fiber serves to bulk and soften stool. When initiating fiber, it should be titrated up slowly as to not cause abdominal cramping and bloating. Patients may require fiber supplementation to reach the recommended

25 to 30 g daily. Patients with slow transit constipation or refractory pelvic floor dyssynergia do not respond well to high fiber, which should be minimized in this particular group.

Biofeedback

Biofeedback is an effective treatment option for patients with constipation caused by outlet obstruction, particularly dyssynergic defecation. During anorectal biofeedback, patients are trained to use breathing techniques with relaxation of the pelvic floor muscles to produce a propulsive force that facilitates effective evacuation.

PHARMACOLOGIC MANAGEMENT OF CONSTIPATION

When lifestyle, dietary changes, and nonpharmacologic interventions are not enough to ameliorate symptoms, a variety of over-the-counter and prescription medications are available to remedy constipation (**Table 2**).

Table 2
Pharmacologic agents for constipation

Class	Mechanism	Examples
Fiber	Increases the water absorbency properties of stool. Insoluble fiber resists bacterial degradation in the colon and can retain more water than soluble fiber	Bran, psyllium, inulin, methylcellulose, calcium polycarophil
Stimulant laxatives	Directly stimulate mucosa or myenteric plexus to trigger peristaltic contractions and inhibit water absorption	Senna, Bisacodyl, castor oil
Stool softeners	Enhance interaction of stool and water	Docusate
Osmotic laxatives	Create an osmotic gradient caused by poorly absorbed ions and molecules, drawing water into the intestinal lumen that results in soft stool and increased intestinal transit	Polyethylene glycol, lactulose Sorbitol, sodium phosphate, magnesium phosphate
Lubricants	Decrease water absorption and soften stool, allowing easier passage	Mineral oil
Chloride-channel activators	Selectively activate enterocyte type 2 chloride channels, resulting in chloride secretion into the intestinal lumen followed by passive diffusion of sodium and water	Lubiprostone
GC-C activators	Stimulate intestinal epithelial cell GC-C receptors, which increases chloride and bicarbonate secretion and fluid secretion and accelerates stool transit	Linaclotide
Serotonin agents	Stimulate intestinal secretion and motility through activation of 5-Hydroxytryptamine receptor 4 receptors of the enteric nervous system within the gastrointestinal tract	Cisapride, Tegaserod, prucalapride

Abbreviation: GC-C, guanylate cyclase C.

Bulk Fiber

Fiber and fiber supplements (eg, bran, psyllium, methylcellulose, inulin, calcium poly-carbophil) increase the water absorbency properties of stool, stool bulk, consistency, stool weight,[6] and intraluminal volume. Fiber is subject to bacterial fermentation that produces short-chain fatty acids that increase luminal osmolarity and water retention, potentiating the effect on laxation. Common side effects are bloating and flatulence. Fiber is not effective for everyone; it may worsen constipation symptoms in patients with slow transit constipation or refractory outlet dysfunction.

Stimulant Laxatives

Stimulant laxatives act by directly stimulating the mucosa or myenteric plexus on contact that triggers high-amplitude peristaltic contractions and by inhibiting water absorption to increase intestinal motility. Side effects include bothersome abdominal cramping and pain that limit their use and electrolyte abnormalities.

Stool Softeners

Stool softeners act as detergents to enhance interaction between stool and water, which promotes softer stool consistency and facilitates evacuation of hard stool.

Lubricants

Mineral oil is the most commonly used lubricant laxative. This agent decreases water absorption and will soften stool, allowing easier passage. Anal seepage of oily material is common, and lipoid pneumonia can occur if the material is aspirated.

Osmotic Laxatives

Osmotic agents, both saline and hyperosmotic types, create an osmotic gradient through the action of poorly absorbed ions and molecules that are not absorbed in the small bowel but metabolized in the colon. This results in luminal water retention and thus an increase in stool water content, which leads to softer stool and increased intestinal transit.[14] Side effects include abdominal bloating, flatulence, cramping, and distention. These agents are generally well tolerated for long-term use.[15]

Chloride-Channel Activator

Lubiprostone is the sole available agent in this class available by prescription. Chloride-channel activation selectively activates enterocyte type 2 chloride channels, resulting in chloride secretion into the intestinal lumen followed by passive diffusion of sodium and water. The sum effect is an increase in stool water, bowel distention, peristalsis, and laxation without a direct effect on smooth muscle.[16] Side effects are nausea (30%), headache, and diarrhea.[17] Subjects older than 65 experienced fewer and less-severe side effects with lubiprostone than did younger patients.[18]

Guanylate Cyclase C Activator

Linaclotide is the only available agent in this class available by prescription. Linaclotide selectively stimulates intestinal epithelial cell guanylate cyclase C (GC-C) receptors, resulting in an increase in intracellular and extracellular cyclic guanosine monophosphate (cGMP). The net luminal effect is increased chloride and bicarbonate secretion, increased fluid secretion, accelerated stool transit, and laxation.[19] Linaclotide also ameliorates visceral hypersensitivity through a mechanism believed to be dependent on GC-C/cGMP.[20] Evidence indicates that cGMP fluxes out of the epithelial cells into the serosal space to act on the submucosal afferent pain fibers to suppress the nerve firing rate.[21]

Serotonin Agonists

Serotonin agonists stimulate intestinal secretion and motility through activation of 5-hydroxytryptamine receptor 4 receptors of the enteric nervous system within the gastrointestinal tract. Some have been discontinued or restricted (cisapride, Tegaserod) because of potentially harmful cardiovascular side effects. Prucalapride is currently available in Europe and Canada.

SUMMARY

Constipation is a common disorder across all age groups encountered in clinical practice. The prevalence increases significantly with age. It reduces quality of life and imposes a large economic burden on individuals and the health system. As sedentary lifestyle and low-fiber diets contribute to constipation, treatment typically includes increased physical activity, high-fiber diets, and bowel management techniques to facilitate evacuation. However, fiber can worsen some types of chronic constipation. Limited testing will identify the specific type of constipation and could be used if the information gained is apt to alter treatment. Not all patients require the same diagnostic approach. A variety of medications with unique mechanisms of action are available to treat constipation.

REFERENCES

1. Bharucha AE, Dorn SD, Lembo A, et al. American Gastroenterological Association medical position statement on constipation. Gastroenterology 2013;144(1): 211–7.
2. Higgins PD, Johanson JF. Epidemiology of constipation in North America: a systematic review. Am J Gastroenterol 2004;99(4):750–9.
3. Dennison C, Prasad M, Lloyd A, et al. The health-related quality of life and economic burden of constipation. Pharmacoeconomics 2005;23(5):461–76.
4. Longstreth GF, Thompson WG, Chey WD, et al. Functional bowel disorders. Gastroenterology 2006;130(5):1480–91.
5. Foxx-Orenstein AE, McNally MA, Odunsi ST. Update on constipation: one treatment does not fit all. Cleve Clin J Med 2008;75(11):813–24.
6. Gallegos-Orozco JF, Foxx-Orenstein AE, Sterler SM, et al. Chronic constipation in the elderly. Am J Gastroenterol 2012;107(1):18–25 [quiz: 26].
7. Ness J, Hoth A, Barnett MJ, et al. Anticholinergic medications in community-dwelling older veterans: prevalence of anticholinergic symptoms, symptom burden, and adverse drug events. Am J Geriatr Pharmacother 2006;4(1):42–51.
8. Traube M, McCallum RW. Calcium-channel blockers and the gastrointestinal tract. American College of Gastroenterology's Committee on FDA related matters. Am J Gastroenterol 1984;79(11):892–6.
9. Rao SS, Singh S. Clinical utility of colonic and anorectal manometry in chronic constipation. J Clin Gastroenterol 2010;44(9):597–609.
10. Diamant NE, Kamm MA, Wald A, et al. AGA technical review on anorectal testing techniques. Gastroenterology 1999;116(3):735–60.
11. Saad RJ, Hasler WL. A technical review and clinical assessment of the wireless motility capsule. Gastroenterol Hepatol (N Y) 2011;7(12):795–804.
12. Fletcher JG, Busse RF, Riederer SJ, et al. Magnetic resonance imaging of anatomic and dynamic defects of the pelvic floor in defecatory disorders. Am J Gastroenterol 2003;98(2):399–411.

13. Bharucha AE, Pemberton JH, Locke GR 3rd, et al. Gastroenterological Association technical review on constipation. Gastroenterology 2013;144(1):218–38.
14. Xing JH, Soffer EE. Adverse effects of laxatives. Dis Colon Rectum 2001;44(8): 1201–9.
15. Ford AC, Suares NC. Effect of laxatives and pharmacological therapies in chronic idiopathic constipation: systematic review and meta-analysis. Gut 2011;60(2): 209–18.
16. Lacy BE, Levy LC. Lubiprostone: a novel treatment for chronic constipation. Clin Interv Aging 2008;3(2):357–64.
17. Lacy BE, Chey WD. Lubiprostone: chronic constipation and irritable bowel syndrome with constipation. Expert Opin Pharmacother 2009;10(1):143–52.
18. Barish CF, Drossman D, Johanson JF, et al. Efficacy and safety of lubiprostone in patients with chronic constipation. Dig Dis Sci 2010;55(4):1090–7.
19. Harris LA, Crowell MD. Linaclotide, a new direction in the treatment of irritable bowel syndrome and chronic constipation. Curr Opin Mol Ther 2007;9(4):403–10.
20. Johnston JM, Kurtz CB, Macdougall JE, et al. Linaclotide improves abdominal pain and bowel habits in a phase IIb study of patients with irritable bowel syndrome with constipation. Gastroenterology 2010;139(6):1877–86.e2.
21. Silos-Santiago I, Hannig G, Eutamene H, et al. Gastrointestinal pain: unraveling a novel endogenous pathway through uroguanylin/guanylate cyclase-C/cGMP activation. Pain 2013;154(9):1820–30.

Colorectal Cancer and the Elderly

Lukejohn W. Day, MD[a],*, Fernando Velayos, MD, MPH[b]

KEYWORDS

- Colorectal cancer • Colonoscopy • Screening • Surveillance • Elderly • Very elderly
- Adverse events • Quality

KEY POINTS

- Colorectal cancer and adenomas are common in the elderly.
- Colorectal cancer screening can be beneficial to patients, but at some ages and under certain circumstances the harm of screening outweighs the benefits.
- Increasing adverse events, poorer bowel preparation, and more numerous incomplete examinations are observed in older patients undergoing colonoscopy for diagnostic, screening, and surveillance purposes.
- Decisions regarding screening, surveillance, and treatment of colorectal cancer require a multidisciplinary approach that accounts not only for the patient's age, but their health status, preferences, and functional status.

INTRODUCTION

Colorectal cancer is the third leading cancer diagnosed and cause of cancer-related deaths in the United States. In 2013, nearly 143,000 people will be diagnosed with colorectal cancer, 51,000 of whom will die of the disease.[1] Age is an important risk factor in the development of colorectal cancer, with its incidence doubling each successive decade between the ages of 40 and 80 years.[2]

Colorectal cancer disproportionately affects the elderly, necessitating the need for screening and surveillance in this group. However, screening and surveillance decisions in the elderly can be challenging. For example, the definition of elderly based on age alone may not properly capture the appropriateness of screening in an individual. The World Health Organization defines elderly as persons older than 65, yet it is well known that persons of this age are a heterogeneous group, ranging from people of sound health with a long life expectancy to those with multiple comorbid medical conditions, declining cognitive function, and impaired functional status.

Funding: None.
Conflicts of Interest: None.
[a] Division of Gastroenterology, Department of Medicine, San Francisco General Hospital and Trauma Center, 1001 Potrero Avenue, 3D-5, San Francisco, CA 94110, USA; [b] Division of Gastroenterology, Department of Medicine, University of California, San Francisco, San Francisco, CA, USA
* Corresponding author.
E-mail address: lukejohn.day@ucsf.edu

This review addresses several of the complexities and challenges in colorectal cancer screening and surveillance in this rapidly growing and heterogeneous population. First, the authors review the epidemiology and clinical presentation of colorectal cancer in the elderly, and how it differs from that in younger patients. Second, the efficacy of screening modalities and the safety of colonoscopy in the elderly are reviewed. Lastly, data regarding when not to screen a patient based on age is discussed.

EPIDEMIOLOGY

Colorectal cancer is common in the elderly and steadily becomes more frequent as one ages. Approximately 90% of new colorectal cancers are diagnosed in patients older than 50 years (**Fig. 1**).[1] The median age of patients diagnosed with colorectal cancer in the United States is 69 years. Under the age of 65 the incidence of colon cancer is low, at 11.4 per 100,000 persons, but this increases exponentially to 176.1 per 100,000 persons in people older than 65, a trend that is mirrored between both sexes and all racial backgrounds with respect to age.[1] Similar observations are noted with regards to rectal cancer (**Fig. 2**).

Precancerous adenomatous polyps and advanced adenomatous polyps (polyp size ≥10 mm, villous/tubulovillous histologic features, high-grade dysplasia) all have an increased prevalence and incidence in relation to age.[3–5] Prevalence of adenoma and advanced adenoma in persons 70 to 75 years of age double that of persons 40 to 49 years old (**Box 1**).[3,6,7]

Age seems to play a role in several other factors related to polyps. Larger-sized polyps and more right-sided polyps are found in older patients.[8] Moreover, older men have a greater prevalence of adenomatous polyps than older women.

The presentation of colorectal cancer is similar in younger and older patients, although there is a greater detection of proximal cancer in older patients[5] and older patients may be less likely to present with no symptoms.[9,10] Although no one presenting symptom predominates in elderly patients, it should be recognized that elderly patients may have a more subtle presentation, such as vague abdominal pain or a new anemia. Such symptoms cannot be attributed to other causes, and deserve a thorough cancer evaluation in the elderly (**Box 2**).

The recurrence of adenomas and colorectal cancer after diagnosis during colonoscopy does not seem to be influenced by age. Numerous studies have consistently demonstrated that adenomatous polyp recurrence is not affected by patients' age,[11–13] with only one study showing a slight increase in polyp recurrence with age.[14] Instead other factors such an index polyp size (polyp ≥1 cm),[12] number of

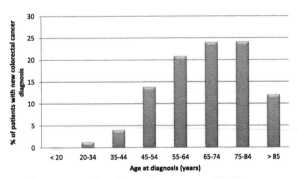

Fig. 1. Distribution of patients with colorectal cancer stratified by age.

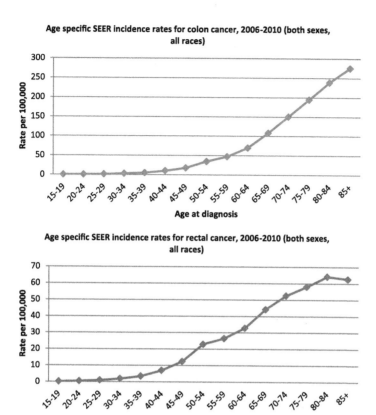

Fig. 2. Incidence rates for colon and rectal cancer for all races and both sexes from 2006 to 2010. SEER, Surveillance Epidemiology and End Results. (*Data from* Howlader N, Noone AM, Krapcho M, et al, editors. SEER cancer statistics review, 1975-2010. Bethesda (MD): National Cancer Institute. Available at: http://seer.cancer.gov/csr/1975_2010/. Accessed July 20, 2013.)

polyps at index colonoscopy,[15] or initial incomplete polyp resection[16] are all more strongly associated with recurrence. With respect to advanced adenomas, similar predictors of recurrence are present, with limited data showing that age may play a role. Two meta-analyses[17,18] examined the recurrence of advanced adenomas after an initial colonoscopy, and discovered that, again, the number of polyps, size of polyps, and polyp histology were strongly associated with the detection of advanced adenoma on a surveillance colonoscopy, with only one of the studies[17] showing that age was a predictor. Recently, a large study from the Netherlands demonstrated

Box 1			
Prevalence of adenomas and advanced adenomas by age group			
Adenoma		**Advanced Adenoma**	
40–49 years	8.7%	40–49 years	1.1%
50–59 years	12.5%	50–59 years	2.4%–5.7%
60–69 years	15.5%	60–69 years	6.6%
70–75 years	25.0%	70–75 years	10.6%–13.0%

Box 2
Presentation of colorectal cancer in the elderly

- Asymptomatic
- Occult blood loss
- Microcytic anemia
- Rectal bleeding
- Change in stool caliber/bowel habits
- Abdominal pain
- Weight loss/cachexia
- Signs of bowel obstruction
- Peritoneal signs/signs of perforation

---

that in addition to polyp size, several other factors relating to polyp and colonoscopy characteristics are associated with the detection of recurrent advanced colorectal neoplasia (advanced adenoma or colorectal cancer) at surveillance colonoscopy (**Box 3**).[15]

Along the same lines, while colorectal cancer incidence increases with age, its recurrence does not seem to be influenced by age. Rather, several other factors listed in **Box 4** have a stronger association.

Given that age does not influence the recurrence of either polyps or colorectal cancer, surveillance guidelines have not been tailored by age.

SCREENING MODALITIES FOR COLORECTAL CANCER

Colorectal cancer screening can detect both precancerous polyps and colorectal cancer, which can lead to a reduction in both incidence and deaths.[19–29] Through screening the incidence of colorectal cancer can be reduced by 17% to 33%, with a mortality reduction of 11% to 53% depending on the modality used. Although no single screening method is preferred in the United States, numerous consensus documents have been put forth offering several screening recommendations, including those from the United States Preventive Services Task Force (USPSTF),[30] the American Cancer Society and the US Multi-Society Taskforce with the American College of Radiology,[31] and the American College of Gastroenterology.[32] Available and recommended screening tests include examining stool for occult blood, radiologic and endoscopic methods (**Box 5**). It should be noted that no one test has been proved to be superior for colorectal cancer screening in the elderly.

Box 3
Predictors of detecting advanced neoplasia at surveillance colonoscopy (based on characteristics from index colonoscopy)

Number of adenomas

Size 1 cm or larger

Villous histology on pathology

Insufficient bowel preparation

Incomplete examination (unable to reach farther than the distal colon)

Box 4
Factors increasing colorectal cancer recurrence

Family history of colorectal cancer

Presence of extracolonic malignancy

Detection of synchronous lesions

Coexisting adenomas

Perforation at time of diagnosis

Symptoms

COLONOSCOPY IN ELDERLY PATIENTS

Rates of colorectal cancer screening in the United States have been steadily rising over the last 20 years, in large part because of the increase in the use of colonoscopy for screening.[33] As more elderly patients undergo colorectal cancer screening using colonoscopy, one has to consider how specific factors related to the procedure and age may interact.

Several reviews[34–36] and a consensus guideline from the American Society of Gastrointestinal Endoscopy[37] have addressed multiple issues regarding the elderly and endoscopy. Very few changes, if any, are recommended for elderly patients with respect to the preprocedure process and sedation. However, 2 differences are noteworthy. First, in elderly patients it is recommended that providers assess for patient's cognitive ability and capacity to understand the procedure, and fully document functional status and depression screening during the preprocedure assessment.[37,38] Second, fewer sedative medications, at lower doses and using medications at slower infusion rates, should be used in the sedation of an elderly patient.[37] Lastly, with the increasing use of general anesthesia in colonoscopy,[39] it should be noted that patients 70 years and older with a greater number of comorbid medical conditions have many more adverse events during colonoscopy when it is performed with the assistance of general anesthesia.[40]

Adverse Events

The occurrence of adverse events during colonoscopy and how age may modify this risk are important considerations for the elderly patient. Age does not play a role in

---

Box 5
Colorectal cancer screening tests

Occult blood

   Guaiac (fecal occult blood test)

   Fecal immunochemical test

Endoscopy

   Colonoscopy

   Flexible sigmoidoscopy

Radiology

   Double-contrast barium enema

   Computed tomographic colonography

---

minor adverse events such as bloating and abdominal pain,[41] but major adverse events such as perforation, bleeding, and cardiopulmonary events (**Boxes 6** and **7**) are all affected by age; however, the individual risk varies and can be influenced by additional factors. Of all adverse events associated with colonoscopy, the major one associated with age is perforation. Patients 65 years or older have a 30% higher risk than younger patients undergoing colonoscopy, and a 14-fold higher risk than patients of the same age who do not undergo the procedure, with the risk being even higher in patients older than 80.[42]

Bowel Preparation

Bowel preparation is a key issue to consider in patients undergoing colonoscopy, as poorer bowel preparations can lead to missed polyps and cancers. Of the 2 agents available (polyethylene glycol electrolyte lavage solution [PEG] and oral sodium phosphate [OSP]), PEG is the preferred agent in older patients. PEG has a better safety profile than OSP, whereby elderly patients are at significantly greater risk of experiencing electrolyte disturbances[43,44] and developing acute kidney injury when taking OSPs.[8,45] The safety profile of each bowel preparation with respect to the elderly is enumerated in **Box 8**.

However, there are concerns with PEG as regards tolerability and compliance in the elderly, with noncompliance rates of 3% to 32%.[46] Moreover, concerns remain with respect to the elderly being able to tolerate such a large volume of fluid required with PEG. Although split PEG-dosing regimens have been shown to be equally effective[47] as standard one-time dosing, this approach has not been studied in the elderly. Of critical importance is that elderly patients remain adequately hydrated when taking PEG.[48]

In addition to determining the optimal and safest bowel preparation for elderly patients, it is equally important to achieve adequate bowel preparation. There is wide variation in documented poor bowel preparations in elderly patients undergoing colonoscopy, ranging from 4% to 57%.[10,49–57] However, adequate bowel preparation seems to be more difficult to achieve in very elderly patients (≥80 years) regardless of whether they are compliant with or of the type of bowel preparation used.[51,55] There are variety of reasons for poorer bowel preparations in the elderly (**Box 9**).

Completion of Colonoscopy

Adequate bowel preparation is key to high-quality colonoscopy, but just as important is the successful completion of a colonoscopy (ie, intubation of the cecum). Endoscopists subjectively judge a colonoscopy to be more difficult in an elderly patient,[58] but completion rates vary from 78% to 86% in the elderly and from 52% to 95%[49,50,59] in the very elderly.[10,51–53,55–57] Mixed data indicate that age may be an independent risk factor for lower completions rates, but it is apparent that other factors such as

Box 6 Adverse events during colonoscopy (≥65 years)	
Adverse Event	**Incidence Rate (per 100,000)**
All major adverse events	26.0
Perforation	1.0
Bleeding	6.3
Cardiopulmonary	19.1
Mortality	1.0

Box 7 Adverse events during colonoscopy (≥80 years)	
Adverse Event	**Incidence Rate (per 100,000)**
All major adverse events	34.9
Perforation	1.5
Bleeding	2.4
Cardiopulmonary	28.9
Mortality	0.5

poor bowel preparation and a patient's underlying disease process play a stronger role.[49,60]

DECISIONS REGARDING NOT SCREENING AND NOT TREATING COLORECTAL CANCER

One of the issues that must be addressed when discussing the elderly, colorectal cancer, and screening is the role of comorbid medical conditions. Elderly patients have a greater number and severity of comorbid medical conditions; more than one-quarter of patients 65 years and older have more than 5 comorbid medical conditions, with a mean of 3.5.[61] Such an increase in comorbid medical conditions can play a role in developing colorectal cancer, and reduce the benefit from screening and treatment. Patients with a diagnosis of colorectal cancer have a greater number of comorbid medical conditions,[62,63] with some conditions, such as obesity and diabetes, having a significant impact on the risk of developing colorectal cancer.[64] It is clear that the benefit of screening is reduced with increasing disease burden. Ko and Sonnenberg[65] showed that the greatest number needed to screen to prevent a colorectal cancer death was in older, more ill patients, and that screening-related complications were greater than the benefit in that cohort. In addition, complications related to colonoscopy (including screening) increase as the number of comorbid medical conditions also increases.[66] Lastly, patients with a greater number of comorbid medical conditions have lower survival rates after an initial diagnosis of colorectal cancer,[67–69] poorer survival after chemotherapy,[69,70] and more prolonged hospitalizations as a consequence of their colorectal cancer.[71,72]

Box 8 Adverse events associated with bowel preparation in elderly patients	
Polyethylene Glycol	**Oral Sodium Phosphate**
Dizziness (48%)	Hyperphosphatemia (58.1%–100%)
Fecal incontinence (27%–39%)	Fecal incontinence (23%–55%)
Abdominal pain (7%–23%)	Elevated creatinine/renal injury (55.2%)
Nausea (2%–17.5%)	Hypocalcemia (5.1%–58%)
Insomnia (13%)	Hypokalemia (5.4%–56%)
Fatigue (12.7%)	Abdominal pain (11%–32%)
Headache (7.9%)	Nausea (9%–36%)
Hypokalemia (2.9%–20.5%)	Insomnia (15%)
Dysnatremia (hyponatremia/ hypernatremia) (4.1%)	Dizziness (3%–55%)
Emesis (3.2%)	Emesis (4%–7%)
Aspiration pneumonia (<1%)	Hypotension (4%)
Pancreatitis (<1%)	
Ischemic colitis (<1%)	

Box 9
Explanations for poorer bowel preparations in the elderly
Altered gastrointestinal motility leading to slower colonic transit time
Increased rates of constipation due to medications
History of previous surgery
Decreased understanding of bowel preparation instructions
Greater burden of comorbid medical conditions
Functional limitations

While detecting colorectal cancer earlier is beneficial the question that remains is does it extend life in older patients who may have a shorter life expectancy? As one ages, and especially in older age groups, life expectancy decreases. For example in the U.S. in 2007 a person at 65 years of age had 18.6 years of life expectancy compared to a person at age 75 years who had only 11.7 years.[72] This raises the question at what point does colorectal cancer screening cease to provide an important potential extension in life expectancy and therefore not be offered?

Several groups have attempted to answer this question from 2 perspectives: (1) gain in life expectancy through screening, and (2) the age at which screening does not provide additional benefit to the patient. On the first question, Inadomi and Sonnenberg[73] conducted modeling studies examining the impact of various colorectal screening methods on life expectancy at different ages. Younger patients had a much more significant decrease in life expectancy than did elderly patients after a diagnosis of colorectal cancer. Simultaneously, for each colorectal cancer screening method there was a nearly 75% reduction in the benefit of screening for elderly patients when compared with younger patients (**Box 10**). These results have been confirmed in similar studies.[74,75] Furthermore, the benefit of screening, in particular colonoscopy, after an initial negative screening test is greatly reduced in elderly patients, as older patients will overwhelmingly succumb to other illnesses (cardiovascular, pulmonary, extracolonic malignancies) rather than colorectal cancer itself.[67] Along the same lines, in a recent study of patients older than 70 years with a positive fecal occult blood test, 46% of the patients who did not undergo colonoscopy died of other causes. Of those who underwent colonoscopy, 10% experienced an adverse event and 86% with a worse life expectancy did not benefit from screening.[76]

As to the second question, multiple studies have examined various ages at which to discontinue colorectal cancer screening. Decreasing the screening age from 85 to 75 years yields small reductions in life years gained and uses fewer resources. Stopping screening at 75 provides almost the same benefit as stopping at 85 years.[77]

Box 10		
Impact of colorectal cancer screening on life expectancy		
	Ages 50–54 (days)	Ages 70–74 (days)
Decrease in life expectancy from colorectal diagnosis	292	70
Increase in life expectancy using fecal occult blood test	51	12
Increase in life expectancy using flexible sigmoidoscopy	86	21
Increase in life expectancy using colonoscopy	170	41

Others have demonstrated diminishing returns for days of life lost after the age of 70 for any form of screening,[78] and that after the age of 60 the percentage of life years saved declines precipitously after a single colonoscopy.[74]

In addition, there does appear to be an age beyond which some patients achieve no benefit from screening. Men 85 years and older, and women 90 years and older, do not achieve any benefit from colorectal cancer screening regardless of modality,[65] and patients older than 80 years have a shortened life expectancy (median survival of <5 years) after a diagnosis of colorectal cancer, regardless of comorbid medical conditions or functional status.[67] However, there is very little guidance from national medical societies on when to stop screening, as **Box 11** illustrates. In summary, most agree that health and functional status, as well as age, should all play a role in deciding when to discontinue screening.

TREATMENT

Once a patient is diagnosed with colorectal cancer, concerns arise about the ability of elderly patients to tolerate and derive benefit from treatment. Several reviews have addressed colorectal cancer treatment and the elderly.[79] Unfortunately, much of the data on chemotherapy for colorectal cancer and the elderly are limited, as advanced age is an exclusion factor in many clinical trials.[79–82] In fact, in many cases, oncologists reduce the dose of chemotherapy for perceived risks of impaired liver or renal function in older patients.[83] Nevertheless, given these limitations and despite theoretical concerns, it does appear that most chemotherapeutic agents are safe in elderly patients and can achieve the same therapeutic benefits of reduced recurrence and mortality as observed in younger patients, especially in the adjuvant setting.[84,85] Given

---

Box 11
Colorectal cancer screening guidelines and the elderly

Society	Recommendation
US Multi-Society Task Force and the American Cancer Society (USMSTF/ACS)	In those with a prior polyp: Discontinuation of surveillance colonoscopy should be considered in persons with serious comorbidities and with less than 10 years of life expectancy
American Gastroenterological Association (AGA)	No comment on when to stop screening. Comment on need for shared decision making and individualized approach
American Geriatrics Society (AGS)	Not recommended in those unlikely to live more than 5 years or who have significant comorbidity that would preclude treatment
British Society of Gastroenterology	Fecal occult blood test every 2 years offered to all persons 50 to 69 years of age (depending on location) with current plans to extend to age 75 in most areas
Kaiser Permanent Care Management Institute (KPCMI)	Discontinuation of screening is generally recommended at age 75, provided there is a history of routine screening Discontinuation is recommended at age 80 for those with no history of routine screening. The decision to discontinue screening should be based on physician judgment, patient preference, the increased risk of complications in older adults, and existing comorbidities

these data, most researchers advocate that age alone should not be factored into one's decision to treat colorectal cancer.[82,84,86] In most instances, comorbid medical conditions play a larger role in the decision to proceed with chemotherapy, as this has a more pronounced impact on life expectancy after the diagnosis and treatment of colorectal cancer.[69] In the end, oncologists advocate a multidisciplinary approach in treating elderly patients with colorectal cancer. A patient's functional status, comorbid medical conditions, patients' goals and preferences, and cancer stage all have to be factored into the decision of determining which regimen (if any) to use when treating the elderly patient with colorectal cancer.[79,82]

SUMMARY

A large proportion of diagnoses of and deaths from colorectal cancer occur in elderly patients. Advancing age is an independent risk factor associated with both colorectal cancer and adenomas, whereas the detection of recurrent colorectal cancer and adenomas after a screening colonoscopy is unaffected by age. Although no single clinical presentation is characteristic of elderly patients with colorectal cancer, it is recognized that elderly patients present with more symptoms. Several colorectal cancer screening modalities are available for elderly patients, from which they and their primary care provider can choose. However, at specific ages the risks and increased resources may outweigh the benefit of screening in some elderly patients. In addition, patients with a greater number and severity of comorbid medical conditions, as found in elderly patients, derive less benefit from screening. Given these factors, controversy exists over when to discontinue colorectal cancer screening and surveillance in the elderly. The decision to proceed with screening and surveillance requires an individualized assessment of the elderly patient that takes into account the risks and benefits, and balances this against the patient's health, functional status, and preferences. Some aspects of screening, such as with colonoscopy, need to be factored into this decision-making process. Older patients have a higher risk of adverse events during a colonoscopy, poorer bowel preparations leading to more suboptimal examinations, and, possibly, lower completion rates. Lastly, a variety of colorectal cancer treatments are available for elderly patients and, just as with decisions about when to discontinue screening, a patient's functional status, comorbid medical conditions, and goals and preferences all have to be factored into the decision-making process when determining which regimen to offer.

REFERENCES

1. Howlader N, Noone AM, Krapcho M, et al, editors. SEER cancer statistics review, 1975-2010. Bethesda (MD): National Cancer Institute. Available at: http://seer.cancer.gov/csr/1975_2010/. Accessed July 20, 2013.
2. Rabeneck L, El-Serag HB, Davila JA, et al. Outcomes of colorectal cancer in the United States: no change in survival (1986-1997). Am J Gastroenterol 2003;98: 471-7.
3. Lieberman DA, Weiss DG, Bond JH, et al. Use of colonoscopy to screen asymptomatic adults for colorectal cancer. Veterans Affairs Cooperative Study Group 380. N Engl J Med 2000;343:162-8.
4. Khullar SK, DiSario JA. Colon cancer screening. Sigmoidoscopy or colonoscopy. Gastrointest Endosc Clin N Am 1997;7:365-86.
5. Neugut AI, Jacobson JS, De Vivo I. Epidemiology of colorectal adenomatous polyps. Cancer Epidemiol Biomarkers Prev 1993;2:159-76.

6. Strul H, Kariv R, Leshno M, et al. The prevalence rate and anatomic location of colorectal adenoma and cancer detected by colonoscopy in average-risk individuals aged 40-80 years. Am J Gastroenterol 2006;101:255–62.

7. Imperiale TF, Wagner DR, Lin CY, et al. Results of screening colonoscopy among persons 40 to 49 years of age. N Engl J Med 2002;346:1781–5.

8. Singal AK, Rosman AS, Post JB, et al. The renal safety of bowel preparations for colonoscopy: a comparative study of oral sodium phosphate solution and polyethylene glycol. Aliment Pharmacol Ther 2008;27:41–7.

9. Trombold J, Farmer RW, McCafferty M. The impact of colorectal cancer screening in a veteran hospital population. Am Surg 2013;79:296–300.

10. Bat L, Pines A, Shemesh E, et al. Colonoscopy in patients aged 80 years or older and its contribution to the evaluation of rectal bleeding. Postgrad Med J 1992;68:355–8.

11. Noshirwani KC, van Stolk RU, Rybicki LA, et al. Adenoma size and number are predictive of adenoma recurrence: implications for surveillance colonoscopy. Gastrointest Endosc 2000;51:433–7.

12. Harewood GC, Lawlor GO. Incident rates of colonic neoplasia according to age and gender: implications for surveillance colonoscopy intervals. J Clin Gastroenterol 2005;39:894–9.

13. Harewood GC, Lawlor GO, Larson MV. Incident rates of colonic neoplasia in older patients: when should we stop screening? J Gastroenterol Hepatol 2006;21:1021–5.

14. Winawer SJ, Zauber AG, O'Brien MJ, et al. Randomized comparison of surveillance intervals after colonoscopic removal of newly diagnosed adenomatous polyps. The National Polyp Study Workgroup. N Engl J Med 1993;328:901–6.

15. van Heijningen EM, Lansdorp-Vogelaar I, Kuipers EJ, et al. Features of adenoma and colonoscopy associated with recurrent colorectal neoplasia based on a large community-based study. Gastroenterology 2013;144:1410–8.

16. Pohl H, Srivastava A, Bensen SP, et al. Incomplete polyp resection during colonoscopy—results of the complete adenoma resection (CARE) study. Gastroenterology 2013;144:74–80.e1.

17. Martinez ME, Baron JA, Lieberman DA, et al. A pooled analysis of advanced colorectal neoplasia diagnoses after colonoscopic polypectomy. Gastroenterology 2009;136:832–41.

18. Saini SD, Kim HM, Schoenfeld P. Incidence of advanced adenomas at surveillance colonoscopy in patients with a personal history of colon adenomas: a meta-analysis and systematic review. Gastrointest Endosc 2006;64:614–26.

19. Faivre J, Dancourt V, Lejeune C, et al. Reduction in colorectal cancer mortality by fecal occult blood screening in a French controlled study. Gastroenterology 2004;126:1674–80.

20. Hardcastle JD, Chamberlain JO, Robinson MH, et al. Randomised controlled trial of faecal-occult-blood screening for colorectal cancer. Lancet 1996;348:1472–7.

21. Kronborg O, Fenger C, Olsen J, et al. Randomised study of screening for colorectal cancer with faecal-occult-blood test. Lancet 1996;348:1467–71.

22. Lindholm E, Brevinge H, Haglind E. Survival benefit in a randomized clinical trial of faecal occult blood screening for colorectal cancer. Br J Surg 2008;95:1029–36.

23. Mandel JS, Bond JH, Church TR, et al. Reducing mortality from colorectal cancer by screening for fecal occult blood. Minnesota Colon Cancer Control Study. N Engl J Med 1993;328:1365–71.

24. Quintero E, Castells A, Bujanda L, et al. Colonoscopy versus fecal immunochemical testing in colorectal-cancer screening. N Engl J Med 2012;366:697–706.

25. Atkin WS, Edwards R, Kralj-Hans I, et al. Once-only flexible sigmoidoscopy screening in prevention of colorectal cancer: a multicentre randomised controlled trial. Lancet 2010;375:1624–33.

26. Segnan N, Senore C, Andreoni B, et al. Randomized trial of different screening strategies for colorectal cancer: patient response and detection rates. J Natl Cancer Inst 2005;97:347–57.

27. Schoen RE, Pinsky PF, Weissfeld JL, et al. Colorectal-cancer incidence and mortality with screening flexible sigmoidoscopy. N Engl J Med 2012;366:2345–57.

28. Zauber AG, Winawer SJ, O'Brien MJ, et al. Colonoscopic polypectomy and long-term prevention of colorectal-cancer deaths. N Engl J Med 2012;366:687–96.

29. Robertson DJ, Greenberg ER, Beach M, et al. Colorectal cancer in patients under close colonoscopic surveillance. Gastroenterology 2005;129:34–41.

30. U.S. Preventive Services Task Force. Screening for colorectal cancer: U.S. Preventive Services Task Force recommendation statement. Ann Intern Med 2008;149:627–37.

31. Levin B, Lieberman DA, McFarland B, et al. Screening and surveillance for the early detection of colorectal cancer and adenomatous polyps, 2008: a joint guideline from the American Cancer Society, the US Multi-Society Task Force on Colorectal Cancer, and the American College of Radiology. Gastroenterology 2008;134:1570–95.

32. Rex DK, Johnson DA, Anderson JC, et al. American College of Gastroenterology guidelines for colorectal cancer screening 2009 [corrected]. Am J Gastroenterol 2009;104:739–50.

33. Joseph DA, King JB, Miller JW, et al. Prevalence of colorectal cancer screening among adults—Behavioral Risk Factor Surveillance System, United States, 2010. MMWR Morb Mortal Wkly Rep 2012;61(Suppl):51–6.

34. Day LW, Walter LC, Velayos F. Colorectal cancer screening and surveillance in the elderly patient. Am J Gastroenterol 2011;106:1197–206 [quiz: 1207].

35. Travis AC, Pievsky D, Saltzman JR. Endoscopy in the elderly. Am J Gastroenterol 2012;107:1495–501 [quiz: 1494, 1502].

36. Jafri SM, Monkemuller K, Lukens FJ. Endoscopy in the elderly: a review of the efficacy and safety of colonoscopy, esophagogastroduodenoscopy, and endoscopic retrograde cholangiopancreatography. J Clin Gastroenterol 2010;44:161–6.

37. Early DS, Acosta RD, Chandrasekhara V, et al. Modifications in endoscopic practice for the elderly. Gastrointest Endosc 2013;78:1–7.

38. Chow WB, Rosenthal RA, Merkow RP, et al. Optimal preoperative assessment of the geriatric surgical patient: a best practices guideline from the American College of Surgeons National Surgical Quality Improvement Program and the American Geriatrics Society. J Am Coll Surg 2012;215:453–66.

39. Liu H, Waxman DA, Main R, et al. Utilization of anesthesia services during outpatient endoscopies and colonoscopies and associated spending in 2003-2009. JAMA 2012;307:1178–84.

40. Cooper GS, Kou TD, Rex DK. Complications following colonoscopy with anesthesia assistance: a population-based analysis. JAMA Intern Med 2013;173:551–6.

41. Ko CW, Riffle S, Shapiro JA, et al. Incidence of minor complications and time lost from normal activities after screening or surveillance colonoscopy. Gastrointest Endosc 2007;65:648–56.

42. Day LW, Kwon A, Inadomi JM, et al. Adverse events in older patients undergoing colonoscopy: a systematic review and meta-analysis. Gastrointest Endosc 2011;74:885–96.

43. Beloosesky Y, Grinblat J, Weiss A, et al. Electrolyte disorders following oral sodium phosphate administration for bowel cleansing in elderly patients. Arch Intern Med 2003;163:803–8.

44. Caswell M, Thompson WO, Kanapka JA, et al. The time course and effect on serum electrolytes of oral sodium phosphates solution in healthy male and female volunteers. Can J Clin Pharmacol 2007;14:e260–74.

45. Russmann S, Lamerato L, Marfatia A, et al. Risk of impaired renal function after colonoscopy: a cohort study in patients receiving either oral sodium phosphate or polyethylene glycol. Am J Gastroenterol 2007;102:2655–63.

46. Hsu CW, Imperiale TF. Meta-analysis and cost comparison of polyethylene glycol lavage versus sodium phosphate for colonoscopy preparation. Gastrointest Endosc 1998;48:276–82.

47. Cohen LB. Split dosing of bowel preparations for colonoscopy: an analysis of its efficacy, safety, and tolerability. Gastrointest Endosc 2010;72:406–12.

48. Lichtenstein GR, Cohen LB, Uribarri J. Review article: bowel preparation for colonoscopy—the importance of adequate hydration. Aliment Pharmacol Ther 2007;26:633–41.

49. Karajeh MA, Sanders DS, Hurlstone DP. Colonoscopy in elderly people is a safe procedure with a high diagnostic yield: a prospective comparative study of 2000 patients. Endoscopy 2006;38:226–30.

50. Ma WT, Mahadeva S, Kunanayagam S, et al. Colonoscopy in elderly Asians: a prospective evaluation in routine clinical practice. J Dig Dis 2007;8:77–81.

51. Lukens FJ, Loeb DS, Machicao VI, et al. Colonoscopy in octogenarians: a prospective outpatient study. Am J Gastroenterol 2002;97:1722–5.

52. Burtin P, Bour B, Charlois T, et al. Colonic investigations in the elderly: colonoscopy or barium enema? Aging (Milano) 1995;7:190–4.

53. Chatrenet P, Friocourt P, Ramain JP, et al. Colonoscopy in the elderly: a study of 200 cases. Eur J Med 1993;2:411–3.

54. George ML, Tutton MG, Jadhav VV, et al. Colonoscopy in older patients: a safe and sound practice. Age Ageing 2002;31:80–1.

55. Schmilovitz-Weiss H, Weiss A, Boaz M, et al. Predictors of failed colonoscopy in nonagenarians: a single-center experience. J Clin Gastroenterol 2007;41:388–93.

56. Duncan JE, Sweeney WB, Trudel JL, et al. Colonoscopy in the elderly: low risk, low yield in asymptomatic patients. Dis Colon Rectum 2006;49:646–51.

57. Syn WK, Tandon U, Ahmed MM. Colonoscopy in the very elderly is safe and worthwhile. Age Ageing 2005;34:510–3.

58. Ristikankare M, Hartikainen J, Heikkinen M, et al. The effects of gender and age on the colonoscopic examination. J Clin Gastroenterol 2001;32:69–75.

59. Ure T, Dehghan K, Vernava AM 3rd, et al. Colonoscopy in the elderly. Low risk, high yield. Surg Endosc 1995;9:505–8.

60. Nelson DB, McQuaid KR, Bond JH, et al. Procedural success and complications of large-scale screening colonoscopy. Gastrointest Endosc 2002;55:307–14.

61. Yancik R. Cancer burden in the aged: an epidemiologic and demographic overview. Cancer 1997;80:1273–83.

62. Jorgensen TL, Hallas J, Friis S, et al. Comorbidity in elderly cancer patients in relation to overall and cancer-specific mortality. Br J Cancer 2012;106:1353–60.

63. van Leersum NJ, Janssen-Heijnen ML, Wouters MW, et al. Increasing prevalence of comorbidity in patients with colorectal cancer in the South of the Netherlands 1995-2010. Int J Cancer 2013;132:2157–63.

64. Rasool S, Kadla SA, Rasool V, et al. A comparative overview of general risk factors associated with the incidence of colorectal cancer. Tumour Biol 2013;34: 2469–76.

65. Ko CW, Sonnenberg A. Comparing risks and benefits of colorectal cancer screening in elderly patients. Gastroenterology 2005;129:1163–70.

66. Warren JL, Klabunde CN, Mariotto AB, et al. Adverse events after outpatient colonoscopy in the Medicare population. Ann Intern Med 2009;150:849–57 W152.

67. Kahi CJ, Azzouz F, Juliar BE, et al. Survival of elderly persons undergoing colonoscopy: implications for colorectal cancer screening and surveillance. Gastrointest Endosc 2007;66:544–50.

68. van de Poll-Franse LV, Haak HR, Coebergh JW, et al. Disease-specific mortality among stage I-III colorectal cancer patients with diabetes: a large population-based analysis. Diabetologia 2012;55:2163–72.

69. Gross CP, McAvay GJ, Krumholz HM, et al. The effect of age and chronic illness on life expectancy after a diagnosis of colorectal cancer: implications for screening. Ann Intern Med 2006;145:646–53.

70. Stavrou EP, Lu CY, Buckley N, et al. The role of comorbidities on the uptake of systemic treatment and 3-year survival in older cancer patients. Ann Oncol 2012;23:2422–8.

71. Sarfati D, Tan L, Blakely T, et al. Comorbidity among patients with colon cancer in New Zealand. N Z Med J 2011;124:76–88.

72. National Center for Health Statistics, Centers for Disease Control and Prevention. Life expectancy at birth, at 65 years of age, and at 75 years of age, by race and sex: United States, selected years 1900-2007. Available at: www.cdc.gov/nchs. Accessed August 1, 2013.

73. Inadomi JM, Sonnenberg A. The impact of colorectal cancer screening on life expectancy. Gastrointest Endosc 2000;51:517–23.

74. Sonnenberg A, Delco F. Cost-effectiveness of a single colonoscopy in screening for colorectal cancer. Arch Intern Med 2002;162:163–8.

75. Lin OS, Kozarek RA, Schembre DB, et al. Screening colonoscopy in very elderly patients: prevalence of neoplasia and estimated impact on life expectancy. JAMA 2006;295:2357–65.

76. Kistler CE, Kirby KA, Lee D, et al. Long-term outcomes following positive fecal occult blood test results in older adults: benefits and burdens. Arch Intern Med 2011;171:1344–51.

77. Zauber AG, Lansdorp-Vogelaar I, Knudsen AB, et al. Evaluating test strategies for colorectal cancer screening: a decision analysis for the U.S. Preventive Services Task Force. Ann Intern Med 2008;149:659–69.

78. Maheshwari S, Patel T, Patel P. Screening for colorectal cancer in elderly persons: who should we screen and when can we stop? J Aging Health 2008;20:126–39.

79. Feliu J, Sereno M, Castro JD, et al. Chemotherapy for colorectal cancer in the elderly: whom to treat and what to use. Cancer Treat Rev 2009;35:246–54.

80. Yee KW, Pater JL, Pho L, et al. Enrollment of older patients in cancer treatment trials in Canada: why is age a barrier? J Clin Oncol 2003;21:1618–23.

81. Lewis JH, Kilgore ML, Goldman DP, et al. Participation of patients 65 years of age or older in cancer clinical trials. J Clin Oncol 2003;21:1383–9.

82. Leo S, Accettura C, Gnoni A, et al. Systemic treatment of gastrointestinal cancer in elderly patients. J Gastrointest Cancer 2013;44:22–32.

83. Shayne M, Culakova E, Wolff D, et al. Dose intensity and hematologic toxicity in older breast cancer patients receiving systemic chemotherapy. Cancer 2009; 115:5319–28.
84. Dotan E, Browner I, Hurria A, et al. Challenges in the management of older patients with colon cancer. J Natl Compr Canc Netw 2012;10:213–24 [quiz: 225].
85. Sundararajan V, Mitra N, Jacobson JS, et al. Survival associated with 5-fluoro-uracil-based adjuvant chemotherapy among elderly patients with node-positive colon cancer. Ann Intern Med 2002;136:349–57.
86. Balducci L. Geriatric oncology. Crit Rev Oncol Hematol 2003;46:211–20.

Endoscopy in the Elderly
Risks, Benefits, and Yield of Common Endoscopic Procedures

Farid Razavi, MD*, Seth Gross, MD, Seymour Katz, MD

KEYWORDS

- Gastroenterology • Endoscopy • Colonoscopy • Advanced endoscopy • Utility
- Screening

KEY POINTS

- The elderly represent a vastly heterogeneous population with greater variation in health, disease, and debility than any other population group. Tailored approaches to clinical research and recommendations become necessary. Endoscopic procedures are generally well tolerated and being elderly should not be cause for withholding procedures.
- In many cases, the risks of preparation and sedation may be greater than the procedure.
- At the core of the decision to undergo diagnostic or therapeutic endoscopy is a vital discussion regarding personalized risk and benefit.
- In frail patients, the risks of a given procedure may be overshadowed by limited benefits in the setting of shortened life expectancy.

INTRODUCTION

It is well known that human longevity continues to increase and that many individuals defined as elderly, older than the age of 65, are living healthy and full lives and are using gastroenterology services in greater numbers than ever before. The most recent World Health Organization report published life expectancies increasing with greater development, hygiene, and accessible health care throughout the world. In the United States, men and women can expect to reach 76 and 81 years, respectively.[1] The US census bureau estimates that by 2030, the number of people older than the age of 85 will double to 8.9 million and, more impressively, 130,000 centenarians will be counted in that same year.[2] The elderly account for a small but growing fraction of the population but use a tremendous amount of resources, accounting for 30% of primary care visits, 47% of total hospital days, and 60% of total health care expenditure.[3] There has been limited research examining the risks, benefits, and use of common

Division of Gastroenterology, Langone Medical Center, New York University, 550 1st Avenue, New York, NY 10016, USA
* Corresponding author.
E-mail address: razavi.farid@gmail.com

Clin Geriatr Med 30 (2014) 133–147
http://dx.doi.org/10.1016/j.cger.2013.10.010
0749-0690/14/$ – see front matter © 2014 Elsevier Inc. All rights reserved.

endoscopic procedures in the elderly. Furthermore, gastroenterology training programs do not routinely incorporate elderly concerns when dealing with common gastrointestinal (GI) issues.

Although endoscopy has been shown to be generally well tolerated in the elderly, they represent a heterogeneous population.[4] There exists a broad array of endoscopic procedures with varying inherent risks that must be weighed with each elderly patient in mind. Discussion of the benefits and drawbacks of the most common procedures and indications for endoscopy including upper endoscopy, colonoscopy, endoscopic retrograde cholangiopancreatography (ERCP), endoscopic ultrasound (EUS), percutaneous endoscopic gastrostomy (PEG), and deep enteroscopy is indicated but not required. Population screening and surveillance colonoscopy issues in the elderly are paramount and require a separate discussion on shared decision making given the reality of increasing risk and diminishing benefit.

AGE-RELATED CHANGES IN PHYSIOLOGY

Age-related physiologic changes in the GI tract must be addressed. Changes are apparent at the cellular level with regard to replication, cell growth, gut immunology, and differentiation leading to a multitude of disorders including GI malignancies, diverticular disease, and dysmotility.[5] The most common age-related changes are as follows:

- Aspiration pneumonia/pneumonitis[6,7]
  - Declining gag reflex with age
  - Increasing secretions
- Cholelithiasis and choledocolithiasis[8,9]
  - Decreased gallbladder emptying
  - Decreased responsiveness to cholecystokinin[10]
- Gastrointestinal bleeding requiring urgent endoscopy[11]
  - Higher rates of nonsteroidal anti-inflammatory drug use
  - Reduced mucosal protective barriers
  - Measurable age-related changes in the bicarbonate level
  - Loss or reduction of the gel protective layer

Additionally, alterations in physiology including decrements in renal function, hepatic function, and cardiopulmonary function have a dramatic impact on periprocedural risk. It is vital to understand systemic and specific GI changes in physiology because it effects the decision to undergo endoscopic procedures.

PREPROCEDURE ASSESSMENT

Before any procedure, a detailed history and physical assessment should be performed to best assess the patient's comorbidities, degree of debility, ability to consent, and ability to successfully follow preprocedural and postprocedural instruction. In one cross-sectional study including 250 gastroenterologists, 71.1% attributed a lack of fundamental understanding regarding precolonoscopy instructions, which would result in an unsuccessful bowel preparation.[10] There are limited data on cognitive or educational barriers to colonoscopy in the elderly. However, studies extrapolating from the general population suggest that difficulty maintaining the preprocedural diet, preparation, and appropriate medication discontinuation are major issues that need to be addressed.[10]

Obtaining an accurate medication history with special emphasis on over-the-counter medications, anticoagulants, and antiplatelet agents is of key importance because many endoscopic procedures involve a higher risk of postprocedural bleeding, particularly polypectomy, endoscopic mucosal resection, or sphincterotomy.

The elderly have the highest rates of polypharmacy, consuming the greatest amount of prescription medications, over-the-counter drugs, and dietary supplements.[12] Significant gaps in medication reconciliation between hospitals, the community, and long-term care centers create an environment rife with medication recording errors.[13] A large US cohort study concluded that the most frequently missed medications on discharge were cardiovascular medications, accounting for 27% of all medication discrepancies at discharge and less than half of all patients with discrepancies at discharge were alerted appropriately.[14] Monitoring antihypertensive and diuretic use becomes especially important in the setting of bowel preparation with an increased risk of dehydration and periprocedural hypotension. Adverse events related to bowel preparation have been directly linked to use of angiotensin-converting enzyme inhibitors, angiotensin-receptor blockers, diuretics, and nonsteroidal anti-inflammatory drugs.[15] Oral antihyperglycemics should not be taken on the morning of the procedure. Long-acting insulin formulations should be halved and early morning procedures are preferred given the increased risk of hypoglycemia in this population. A thorough reconciliation of all medications is essential.

BOWEL PREPARATION

Colonoscopy bowel preparation adds a potential physiologic challenge for the elderly patient. In the very elderly population, several large studies have shown successful colonic preparation is more difficult to achieve despite patient compliance, tolerance, and the type of preparation used.[16–18] Poor preparation may be related to redundant colon length, intolerance to the volume of preparation, decreased autonomic innervation of the bowel, and colonic tortuosity. Another concern is the urgency with fecal incontinence and a higher risk of falls and fractures while getting to the bathroom, an event that can be avoided with proper planning and preprocedure assessment.[19] Oral sodium phosphate preparations are associated with a higher risk of electrolyte derangements and phosphate nephropathy in the elderly.[20] A population-based study revealed a significant association between polyethylene glycol preparation and acute renal failure to be most pronounced in the elderly age group.[21] The most likely cause of acute renal failure was related to preprocedure osmotic fluid shifts and subsequent lack of rehydration.

Polyethylene glycol is generally well tolerated in most patient populations, including children and pregnant women. It is the leading choice for bowel preparation in the elderly population despite the large volume load (4 L). The elderly are often uninformed regarding the risks of dehydration and electrolyte imbalance.[15] The elderly are at increased risk for impaired thirst reflex and inadequate renal free water handling, thus hydration is essential before and postprocedure to prevent dysnatremia and renal failure.[15] Split bowel preparation dosing, whereby the patient is instructed to take half the dose the evening before and the remainder on the morning of the examination, has been more successful because of better visualization of the proximal colon and mitigates the risks of noncompliance, fluid shifts, and renal injury in the elderly.[22,23]

SEDATION

Procedural sedation during endoscopy remains relatively safe with minimal complications. The general risks of sedation include decreased respiratory drive, aspiration, and a greater likelihood of endoscopic injury. Several physiologic changes including increased body fat content, compromised renal, and hepatic clearance lead to prolonged recovery and greater risk of oversedation in the elderly.[24] Geriatric patients have a reduction in pharyngeal sensitivity leading to greater risk of aspiration. Therefore airway protection and adequate suction of retained gastric contents during upper endoscopy is paramount. Baseline oxygen tension is lowered in the elderly making supplemental oxygen a necessity during sedation.[24]

Endoscopic sedation has historically used conscious sedation with benzodiazepines (midazolam) and narcotics (fentanyl). However, there has been an increasing trend to using propofol, a short-acting anesthetic agent with monitored anesthesia care.[25] In a large US wide survey, procedural sedation was administered for 98% of upper endoscopies and colonoscopies with 74% using a narcotic and benzodiazepine combination, whereas the remainder used propofol and monitored anesthesia care.[25] Propofol has the benefit of short half-life, quick onset of action, and improved patient tolerance during longer interventional procedures. Despite the overall favorable profile, propofol use requires caution in the elderly given its narrow therapeutic window, lack of reversal agent, and increased risk of cardiopulmonary depression. Two studies revealed a significantly higher likelihood of respiratory depression and arterial hypotension after propofol administration when compared with midazolam in the elderly.[26,27] However, neither study had significantly greater numbers of emergency cardiopulmonary intervention or short- or long-term mortality, suggesting that when used appropriately, propofol is a safe option in the elderly.[26,27]

Another option, sedation-free endoscopy, is reasonable yet often discouraged in the United States; however, most routine endoscopies in Asia and Europe are completed without sedation.[28,29] Data have shown that elderly patients have a higher tolerance and preference for sedation-free procedures.[30,31] A randomized controlled trial by Rex and colleagues[31] revealed that patients receiving sedation on an as-needed basis as opposed to a fixed amount of sedative at the start of a case had a lesser decline in systolic blood pressure and fewer reported cases of hypoxic episodes; additionally, per procedure charges were lower than patients receiving routine sedation. More than 90% of patients randomized to sedation as needed were "very satisfied" and would request the same endoscopist.[31] A recent Veterans Administration study using a water immersion technique revealed pain scores, rates of cecal intubation, and total examination time not to be significantly different between patients given sedation and those who opted against it.[32]

Unsedated endoscopy with an ultrathin scope is yet another option gaining significant traction in the high-risk elderly patient. The ultrathin scope measures 6 mm in diameter compared with the 10- to 11-mm regular endoscope, allowing for ease of passage and less oropharyngeal irritation. A multicenter prospective trial demonstrated the benefits of unsedated ultrathin oral or transnasal endoscopy, which included lower costs, increased patient satisfaction, and shorter procedure times.[33] Yuki and colleagues[34] published a prospective trial comparing ultrathin endoscopy to standard per oral endoscopy in elderly and debilitated patients. They reported significantly decreased rates of oxygen desaturation and cardiopulmonary decompensation as measured by the rate-pressure product (pulse rate × systolic blood pressure/100), which is a good proxy for cardiac stress, when using the ultrathin scope.

UPPER ENDOSCOPY

Several studies have demonstrated the high yield, safety, and effectiveness of upper endoscopy in the elderly population.[35–37] The data suggest that age alone should not be a contraindication for undergoing upper endoscopy. A recent study showed no significant differences in duration of hospital stay, blood transfusion requirements, postendoscopic complications, and in-hospital mortality between the elderly and younger adult patients.[38]

A large retrospective study by Buri and colleagues[35] found predictive factors of GI bleeding, reflux symptoms, weight loss, and dysphagia to be better clinical indications for endoscopy positive findings ranging from 50% to 74%. Asymptomatic patients with family history of gastric cancer, atypical reflux symptoms, and epigastric pain had an endoscopic yield ranging from 6% to 46%.[35]

Despite the relative safety of upper endoscopy, the importance of cardiopulmonary monitoring remains essential because several studies have revealed an increased occurrence of cardiopulmonary events during upper endoscopy in the elderly.[39–42] This must be caused by an aberrant cardiopulmonary reflex pathway between central neural control of the esophagus, lungs, and heart.[43] In one study examining 21,946 endoscopies in the elderly, the occurrence of cardiopulmonary complications in upper endoscopy was 0.04%.[39] Cardiopulmonary events are more frequent in elderly patients with a two-fold increase in those patients with underlying heart disease.[42] Seinelä and colleagues[36] reported a significant increase in premature ventricular contraction frequency in elderly subjects with a pre-existing history of heart disease and periprocedural ST changes. Significant increases in measures of cardiac stress have been reported in the elderly including the rate pressure product[44] and atrial natriuretic peptide.[45] Upper endoscopy with an ultrathin endoscope is an option that has been shown to reduce the likelihood of cardiac stress.[33] Taking a careful cardiac history is an essential component of the pre-endoscopy work-up.

Proper head positioning is crucial when considering the increased risk of aspiration but also in patients with significant cervical arthritis. Intubating the upper esophageal sphincter in elderly patients who are known to have greater risk of having Zenker diverticulum increases the risk of perforation.[46]

COLONOSCOPY

Two large prospective trials and one meta-analysis completed in the last decade have shown diagnostic colonoscopy to be safe and effective for the elderly and very elderly population.[47,48] Arora and colleagues[49] revealed that colonoscopy in patients older than 80 years of age had a significantly higher yield, required significantly less procedural sedation, and had low rates of complications when compared with patients younger than 80 years of age. Considerations that should be factored include procedure times, risk of perforation, and quality of preparation. An increased rate of perforation has been reported in a large retrospective analysis of the California Medicaid claims database. Patients aged older than 80 had a perforation incidence of 115 per 100,000 colonoscopies compared with patients aged 65 to 80 who had 82 per 100,000 colonoscopies ($P = .016$). When age was analyzed more closely in a multivariate analysis, each year conferred a significant additional 1% risk of perforation (odds ratio, 1.01; $P = .007$).[49] The most comprehensive meta-analysis on adverse events in the elderly by Day and colleagues[50] showed the elderly to be at higher risk for several complications, detailed in **Fig. 1**, during and after colonoscopy. The most common complication is cardiopulmonary caused by the effect of procedural sedation rather than the procedure itself. In the very elderly population, there are significantly longer procedure times independent of endoscopist experience.[47] Terminal ileum intubation rates also have been lower.[47] Longer procedure times might be caused by increased colonic tortuosity, redundancy with looping, a higher degree of diverticular disease, and poor colonic preparation making visualization during the examination more difficult.

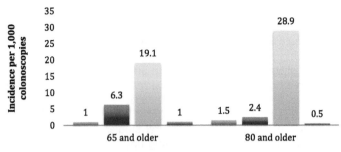

Fig. 1. Major complications during and after colonoscopy in the elderly. (*Data from* Day LW, Kwon A, Inadomi JM, et al. Adverse events in older patients undergoing colonoscopy: a systematic review and meta-analysis. Gastrointest Endosc 2011;74(4):885–96.)

SCREENING COLONOSCOPY IN THE ELDERLY

Rates of colorectal cancer death, the third leading cause of cancer-related death in the United States, have declined rapidly over the last three decades in large part because of the success of successful screening programs and improvements in screening colonoscopy.[51] With the introduction of Medicare coverage for average-risk screening in 2001, the rates of screening colonoscopy have dramatically increased and outpaced barium enema, flexible sigmoidoscopy, and fecal occult blood testing.[52] However, limited research has examined the impact of screening colonoscopy in the elderly. In fact, guidelines written by the American Cancer Society, American College of Gastroenterology, US Multi-Society Task Force on Colorectal Cancer, and American College of Radiology do not discuss or set forth upper age limits on screening.[53] Two recent systematic reviews by the US Preventive Services Task Force and American College of Physicians recommend stopping screening colonoscopy, given limited benefit, beyond the age of 75 (**Box 1**).[54,55] A *New York Times* article signaled a potential shift in public opinion toward decreasing support for screening colonoscopy in the elderly.[56] Medicare claims for Texans older than 70 revealed that 23.4% of colonoscopies performed between 2008 and 2009 were potentially inappropriate, with screenings occurring beyond the recommended age cutoffs and sooner than the recommended 10-year interval.[57–59]

The relative yield of screening colonoscopy in asymptomatic elderly patients remains low. In one retrospective analysis reviewing the indications and yield of 1199

Box 1	
Major society recommendations on when to stop screening	
Society	**Age Limit**
American Cancer Society	No upper age limit
American College of Gastroenterology	No upper age limit
US Multi-Society Task Force on Colorectal Cancer	No upper age limit
American College of Radiology	No upper age limit
US Preventive Services Task Force	75 y
American College of Physicians	75 y

colonoscopies for patients older than 80, none of the patients presenting for screening had a malignancy detected, raising doubts that the oldest elderly patients benefit from continued screening procedures.[60] Patients older than 80 should be referred for colonoscopy only for specific clinical symptoms or findings.

There is lack of communication between primary care physicians, the most common source of screening referral, and their elderly patients regarding the risks of colonoscopy.[61] This issue is prevalent in screening tests in general because recent research has revealed a strong health care system bias toward increasing screening rates rather than careful scrutiny of the risks and benefits for the individual.[62] The success of public health campaigns to increase cancer screening along with a lack of frank communication regarding screening test burdens has led to widespread blind support among many elderly patients.[63] Research focused on adverse events during colonoscopy in the elderly population is scant with most data drawn from studies with mixed populations without significant comorbidities. In one of the first population-based studies to analyze adverse events during screening colonoscopy exclusively in the elderly outpatient population the rate of adverse events including perforation increased significantly by age group and comorbid diseases.[64] Patients with a history of stroke, chronic obstructive pulmonary disease, atrial fibrillation, or congestive heart failure were at significantly increased risk for adverse GI events within 30 days of the procedure.[64]

Given the complexity of risks and benefits involved in colorectal cancer screening decisions, a shared decision-making approach is ideal and has been recommended by the US Preventive Services Task Force.[65] Patient-centered or shared decision making provides an ideal model that empowers and educates patients while promoting trust in the physician-patient relationship. Using a multistep process in which patient and physician freely share data and express their beliefs, patients are able to reach satisfactory informed decisions.[65] Decision making is often aided through the use of well-designed pictographic decision aides as demonstrated in an article by Lewis and colleagues[66] that showed elderly participants to be more knowledgeable, satisfied, and prepared to make an individualized decision. **Fig. 2** provides an example

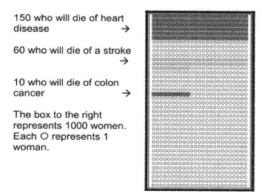

For every 1000 women age 80 there are:

150 who will die of heart disease →

60 who will die of a stroke →

10 who will die of colon cancer →

The box to the right represents 1000 women. Each O represents 1 woman.

Fig. 2. Geriatric decision aid. (*Adapted from* Lewis CL, Golin CE, DeLeon C, et al. A targeted decision aid for the elderly to decide whether to undergo colorectal cancer screening: development and results of an uncontrolled trial. BMC Med Inform Decis Mak 2010;10:54; with permission.)

of the risk-benefit decision aid created specifically for an elderly woman considering screening colonoscopy.

ENDOSCOPIC RETROGRADE CHOLANGIOPANCREATOGRAPHY

Cholelithiasis and choledocolithiasis increase with age.[67] With the successful use of ERCP, higher-risk urgent or emergent surgical procedures can be avoided, leading to significantly lower mortality in the elderly.[68] Therapeutic ERCP in the elderly and very elderly (>85) has been shown to be a safe and cost-effective procedure in inpatients and outpatients.[68–71] In one large prospective observational study, the most common indication for ERCP was biliary obstruction (73.7%).[68] The only significant difference in postprocedure complication rates between patients older than 80 and younger subjects was a greater predilection for hypotension and prolonged sedation.[68] This is suggestive of decreased tolerability of longer procedures and changes in physiologic reserve and drug metabolism in the very elderly. Other complications including acute pancreatitis, intraprocedural bleeding, presence of fever, and abdominal pain were not statistically different between the very elderly and their younger counterparts.[68] Of note, the endoscopies in this study were completed by expert advanced endoscopists, each logging more than 1000 procedures before the start of the study.[72] In another recent prospective trial, including 780 patients, the rates of post-ERCP pancreatitis were shown to be significantly lower in patients older than 70 compared with their younger counterparts.[73] Of interest, there was no significant difference in other complications including perforation, bleeding, and cholangitis.[73] Increasing age may serve as a protectant for postprocedural pancreatitis because the exocrine function of the pancreas diminishes with time.[74]

ENDOSCOPIC ULTRASOUND

EUS has become a standard procedure in cancer staging, evaluation of pancreaticobiliary disease, and subepithelial lesions. However, the echoendoscope has a higher reported risk of complication compared with standard endoscope.[75] This increased risk stems from the increased rigidity of the probe tip and the subsequent risk of perforation. Just as with ERCP, procedure times are longer, exposing patients to increased risks of sedation and cardiopulmonary compromise. There is a general dearth of data regarding the safety and use of EUS in the elderly population. One of the first studies to examine EUS in the elderly population found a similar rate of complications in patients older than 75 years compared with those younger than 75 years.[76] A retrospective analysis of 265 patients with a mean age older than 80 years revealed EUS and EUS with fine-needle aspiration to be safe and well tolerated without complications.[77] Nearly half (48.3%) of all EUS were done to evaluate the pancreas and biliary tree with most of these investigations targeting a specific mass lesion. Other indications for EUS included luminal pathology (30.8%), subepithelial lesions (10.5%), and mediastinal pathology (5.2%). There were no reported cases of EUS-related or EUS with fine-needle aspiration–related perforation or complication.[77]

The combined diagnostic and therapeutic benefits of EUS and ERCP are evident and completion of both in a single session is common. However, there remains very little data on combined procedures in the elderly population. A retrospective study of 206 patients compared the safety of combined ERCP and EUS in the elderly and nonelderly population. Despite significantly higher comorbidity scores in the elderly, there were no significant differences in the incidence of adverse events.[78] Overall, the combination of ERCP and EUS was generally well tolerated and useful for diagnosis and therapeutic intervention.[78]

PERCUTANEOUS ENDOSCOPIC GASTROSTOMY

PEG has become a mainstay for nutritional support in terminally ill and incapacitated patients despite a paucity of quality evidence supporting its use.[79] Few studies have been done examining the impact and safety of PEG placement in the elderly population despite the increased frequency of the procedure in this population. In one retrospective study, the rate of PEG placement in the elderly increased by 38% over a 10-year period between 1993 and 2003 with the leading indications for placement being cerebrovascular disease, aspiration pneumonia, malnutrition, congestive heart failure, and dysphagia.[80] In a prospective cohort study of 150 elderly patients, major complications were rare and no patients died because of PEG placement; however, 70% reported no significant gains in quality of life or functional status.[81] The five most common complications reported included vomiting (30%), diarrhea (26.7%), constipation (22.7%), nausea (20%), and aspiration symptoms (18.7%).[81]

Thirty percent of all PEG tube placements in nursing homes are completed for cognitive impairment or dementia and that number continues to increase.[82] A recent systematic review revealed a significant lack of high-quality research into PEG placement in dementia and failed to show support for prolonged survival, improved quality of life, improved nutrition, or decreased risk of pressure ulcers.[83] In patients with dementia the social interactions that occur during feeding are most important and are ultimately lost with PEG placement.

The difficulty of selecting patients for PEG placement is evidenced by a recent article revealing a robust comprehensive geriatric assessment failed to adequately predict postprocedural mortality.[84] Patients considered for PEG placement should have a life expectancy greater than 30 days.[85]

VIDEOCAPSULE ENDOSCOPY

Small bowel investigation using capsule endoscopy received Food and Drug Administration approval in 2000 and has become an integral part of the work-up of patients with obscure or occult GI bleeding, small intestinal polyps, malignancy, malabsorptive disorders, and inflammatory bowel disease.[86,87] Potential risks include aspiration, capsule retention, and perforation. Few studies have examined the safety and use of the procedure in the elderly population. A retrospective analysis reviewing the safety, tolerability, and findings of capsule endoscopy in the elderly found no significant differences in small bowel transit time or overall safety relative to a matched younger cohort.[88] However, the elderly participants were significantly more likely to label the procedure as tiresome and difficult.[88] The largest cohort study revealed that patients older than 80 were not more likely to suffer adverse events, defined as aspiration or capsule retention, compared with younger participants.[89] Further analysis showed capsule endoscopy to have a higher diagnostic yield in the over 80 population (73%) compared with the younger participants (55%) because of higher frequency of vascular lesions (angiodysplasia).[89] Yet, the detection of polyps, malignancy, and ulceration was no different between age groups.[89] In appropriately selected elderly patients, capsule endoscopy can be considered safe and with a high yield of diagnosis.

DEEP ENTEROSCOPY

Double- and single-balloon enteroscopy have become invaluable tools in the evaluation, diagnosis, and treatment of diseases of the small bowel, namely obscure bleeding. Despite the use, safety, and high yield of deep enteroscopy, few studies have investigated this technique in the elderly population. The most common complications in the general population undergoing deep enteroscopy include perforation, abdominal pain, bleeding, and pancreatitis.[90] A recent prospective review of double-balloon enteroscopy comparing patients older than 70 with those younger revealed a higher yield, significantly lower sedation requirements, and no significant differences in complications between the two groups.[91] Postendoscopy management was modified significantly more often in the elderly.[91] Another retrospective study also revealed a higher diagnostic yield in the elderly with a significantly higher number of small bowel angioectasias and a greater likelihood of requiring endoscopic therapy.[92] Before the advent of deep enteroscopy, many angioectasias were not accessible by standard push enteroscopy and recurrent bleeding required a surgical approach. Deep enteroscopy has become a safe and highly effective tool in the elderly patient.

SUMMARY

With the increasing growth of the elderly population, a refined focus on specific disease states and risk factors is necessary. Although several studies have analyzed the general use and safety of endoscopic procedures including upper endoscopy, colonoscopy, ERCP, and EUS, there is a scarcity of literature focusing exclusively on the elderly. The elderly represent a vastly heterogeneous population with greater variation in health, disease, and debility than any other population group. Tailored approaches to clinical research and recommendations become necessary. Endoscopic procedures are generally well tolerated and being elderly should not be cause for withholding procedures. In many cases, the risks of preparation and sedation may be greater than the procedure. At the core of the decision to undergo diagnostic or therapeutic endoscopy is a vital discussion regarding personalized risk and benefit. In frail patients, the risks of a given procedure may be overshadowed by limited benefits in the setting of shortened life expectancy. Further research on procedure-specific risks in older patients is necessary.

REFERENCES

1. WHO life expectancy tables, 2013. World Health Organization; 2013.
2. Krach C, Velkoff V. Current population reports: special studies, centenarians in the United States. US census bureau 1990. 1999.
3. Hetzel L, Smith A. The 65 years and over population; 2000. US census bureau. 2001.
4. Retrograde E, Jafri S, Monkemuller K, et al. Endoscopy in the elderly a review of the efficacy and safety of colonoscopy, esophagogastroduodenoscopy, and endoscopic retrograde cholangiopancreatography. J Clin Gastroenterol 2010; 44(3):161–6.
5. Camilleri M, Lee JS, Viramontes B, et al. Insights into the pathophysiology and mechanisms of constipation, irritable bowel syndrome, and diverticulosis in older people. J Am Geriatr Soc 2000;48(9):1142–50.
6. Lai PJ, Chen FC, Ho ST, et al. Unexpected pulmonary aspiration during endoscopy under intravenous anesthesia. Acta Anaesthesiol Taiwan 2010;48(2):94–8.
7. Shaker R, Ren J, Bardan E, et al. Pharyngoglottal closure reflex: characterization in healthy young, elderly and dysphagic patients with predeglutitive aspiration. Gerontology 2003;49(1):12–20.
8. Pazzi P, Putinati S, Limone G, et al. The effect of age and sex on gallbladder motor dynamics. An echographic study. Radiol Med 1989;77(4):365–8 [in Italian].
9. Khalil T, Walker JP, Wiener I, et al. Effect of aging on gallbladder contraction and release of cholecystokinin-33 in humans. Surgery 1985;98(3):423–9.

10. Hillyer GC, Basch CH, Basch CE, et al. Gastroenterologists' perceived barriers to optimal pre-colonoscopy bowel preparation: results of a national survey. J Cancer Educ 2012;27(3):526–32.
11. Lee M, Feldman M. The aging stomach: implications for NSAID gastropathy. Gut 1997;41(4):425–6.
12. Gokula M, Holmes HM. Tools to reduce polypharmacy. Clin Geriatr Med 2012; 28(2):323–41.
13. Midlöv P, Bahrani L, Seyfali M, et al. The effect of medication reconciliation in elderly patients at hospital discharge. Int J Clin Pharmacol 2012;34(1):113–9.
14. Unroe KT, Pfeiffenberger T, Riegelhaupt S, et al. Inpatient medication reconciliation at admission and discharge: a retrospective cohort study of age and other risk factors for medication discrepancies. Am J Geriatr Pharmacother 2010;8(2): 115–26.
15. Lichtenstein GR, Cohen LB, Uribarri J. Review article: bowel preparation for colonoscopy–the importance of adequate hydration. Aliment Pharmacol Ther 2007;26(5):633–41.
16. Day LW, Walter LC, Velayos F. Colorectal cancer screening and surveillance in the elderly patient. Am J Gastroenterol 2011;106(7):1197–206 [quiz: 1207].
17. Schmilovitz-Weiss H, Weiss A, Boaz M, et al. Predictors of failed colonoscopy in nonagenarians: a single-center experience. J Clin Gastroenterol 2007;41(4):388–93.
18. Lukens FJ, Loeb DS, Machicao VI, et al. Colonoscopy in octogenarians: a prospective outpatient study. Am J Gastroenterol 2002;97(7):1722–5.
19. Heymann TD, Chopra K, Nunn E, et al. Bowel preparation at home: prospective study of adverse effects in elderly people. BMJ 1996;313(7059):727–8.
20. Rex DK. Dosing considerations in the use of sodium phosphate bowel preparations for colonoscopy. Ann Pharmacother 2007;41(9):1466–75.
21. Choi NK, Lee J, Chang Y, et al. Polyethylene glycol bowel preparation does not eliminate the risk of acute renal failure: a population-based case-crossover study. Endoscopy 2013;45(3):208–13.
22. Hillyer GC, Lebwohl B, Basch CH, et al. Split dose and MiraLAX-based purgatives to enhance bowel preparation quality becoming common recommendations in the US. Therap Adv Gastroenterol 2013;6(1):5–14.
23. Aoun E, Abdul-Baki H, Azar C, et al. A randomized single-blind trial of split-dose PEG-electrolyte solution without dietary restriction compared with whole dose PEG-electrolyte solution with dietary restriction for colonoscopy preparation. Gastrointest Endosc 2005;62(2):213–8.
24. Barnett SR, editor. Manual of geriatric anesthesia. New York: Springer New York; 2013.
25. Cohen LB, Wecsler JS, Gaetano JN, et al. Endoscopic sedation in the United States: results from a nationwide survey. Am J Gastroenterol 2006;101(5): 967–74.
26. Schilling D, Rosenbaum A, Schweizer S, et al. Sedation with propofol for interventional endoscopy by trained nurses in high-risk octogenarians: a prospective, randomized, controlled study. Endoscopy 2009;41(4):295–8.
27. Heuss LT, Schnieper P, Drewe J, et al. Conscious sedation with propofol in elderly patients: a prospective evaluation. Aliment Pharmacol Ther 2003; 17(12):1493–501.
28. Leung FW, Aljebreen AM. Unsedated colonoscopy: is it feasible? Saudi J Gastroenterol 2011;17(4):289–92.
29. Leung FW. The case of unsedated screening colonoscopy in the United States. Gastrointest Endosc 2009;69(7):1354–6.

30. Abraham NS, Fallone CA, Mayrand S, et al. Sedation versus no sedation in the performance of diagnostic upper gastrointestinal endoscopy: a Canadian randomized controlled cost-outcome study. Am J Gastroenterol 2004;99(9):1692–9.

31. Rex DK, Imperiale TF, Portish V. Patients willing to try colonoscopy without sedation: associated clinical factors and results of a randomized controlled trial. Gastrointest Endosc 1999;49(5):554–9.

32. Leung J, Mann S, Siao-Salera R, et al. A randomized, controlled trial to confirm the beneficial effects of the water method on U.S. veterans undergoing colonoscopy with the option of on-demand sedation. Gastrointest Endosc 2011;73(1):103–10.

33. Garcia RT, Cello JP, Nguyen MH, et al. Unsedated ultrathin EGD is well accepted when compared with conventional sedated EGD: a multicenter randomized trial. Gastroenterology 2003;125(6):1606–12.

34. Yuki M, Amano Y, Komazawa Y, et al. Unsedated transnasal small-caliber esophagogastroduodenoscopy in elderly and bedridden patients. World J Gastroenterol 2009;15(44):5586–91.

35. Buri L, Zullo A, Hassan C, et al. Upper GI endoscopy in elderly patients: predictive factors of relevant endoscopic findings. Intern Emerg Med 2013;8(2):141–6.

36. Seinelä L, Ahvenainen J, Rönneikkö J, et al. Reasons for and outcome of upper gastrointestinal endoscopy in patients aged 85 years or more: retrospective study. BMJ 1998;317(7158):575–80.

37. Clarke GA, Jacobson BC, Hammett RJ, et al. The indications, utilization and safety of gastrointestinal endoscopy in an extremely elderly patient cohort. Endoscopy 2001;33(7):580–4.

38. Lee TC, Huang SP, Yang JY, et al. Age is not a discriminating factor for outcomes of therapeutic upper gastrointestinal endoscopy. Hepatogastroenterology 2007;54(77):1319–22.

39. Lee JG, Leung JW, Cotton PB. Acute cardiovascular complications of endoscopy: prevalence and clinical characteristics. Dig Dis 1995;13(2):130–5.

40. Levy N, Abinader E. Continuous electrocardiographic monitoring with Holter electrocardiocorder throughout all stages of gastroscopy. Am J Dig Dis 1977;22(12):1091–6.

41. Lieberman DA, Wuerker CK, Katon RM. Cardiopulmonary risk of esophagogastroduodenoscopy. Role of endoscope diameter and systemic sedation. Gastroenterology 1985;88(2):468–72.

42. McAlpine JK, Martin BJ, Devine BL. Cardiac arrhythmias associated with upper gastrointestinal endoscopy in elderly subjects. Scott Med J 1990;35(4):102–4.

43. Ristikankare M, Julkunen R, Heikkinen M, et al. Cardiac autonomic regulation during gastroscopy. Dig Liver Dis 2009;41(9):648–52.

44. Adachi W, Yazawa K, Owa M, et al. Quantification of cardiac stress during EGD without sedation. Gastrointest Endosc 2002;55(1):58–64.

45. Shimamoto C, Hirata I, Katsu K. Effect of upper gastrointestinal endoscopy on circulation in the elderly. Gerontology 1999;45(4):200–5.

46. De la Mora G, Marcon NE. Endoscopy in the elderly patient. Best Pract Res Clin Gastroenterol 2001;15(6):999–1012.

47. Arora A, Singh P. Colonoscopy in patients 80 years of age and older is safe, with high success rate and diagnostic yield. Gastrointest Endosc 2004;60(3):408–13.

48. Karajeh MA, Sanders DS, Hurlstone DP. Colonoscopy in elderly people is a safe procedure with a high diagnostic yield: a prospective comparative study of 2000 patients. Endoscopy 2006;38(3):226–30.

49. Arora G, Mannalithara A, Singh G, et al. Risk of perforation from a colonoscopy in adults: a large population-based study. Gastrointest Endosc 2009;69(3 Pt 2): 654–64.
50. Day LW, Kwon A, Inadomi JM, et al. Adverse events in older patients undergoing colonoscopy: a systematic review and meta-analysis. Gastrointest Endosc 2011;74(4):885–96.
51. American Cancer Society. Cancer facts and figures 2011. Atlanta (GA): American Cancer Society; 2011.
52. Harewood GC, Lieberman DA. Colonoscopy practice patterns since introduction of Medicare coverage for average-risk screening. Clin Gastroenterol Hepatol 2004;2(1):72–7.
53. Levin B, Lieberman DA, McFarland B, et al. Screening and surveillance for the early detection of colorectal cancer and adenomatous polyps, 2008: a joint guideline from the American Cancer Society, the US Multi-Society Task Force on Colorectal Cancer, and the American College of Radiology. Gastroenterology 2008;134(5):1570–95.
54. Whitlock EP, Lin JS, Liles E, et al. Screening for colorectal cancer: a targeted, updated systematic review for the U.S. Preventive Services Task Force. Ann Intern Med 2008;149(9):638–58.
55. Qaseem A, Denberg TD, Hopkins RH, et al. Screening for colorectal cancer: a guidance statement from the American College of Physicians. Ann Intern Med 2012;156(5):378–86.
56. Too many colonoscopies in the elderly - NYTimes.com. Available at: http://newoldage. blogs.nytimes.com/2013/03/12/too-many-colonoscopies-in-the-elderly/?_r=0. Accessed August 26, 2013.
57. Sheffield KM, Han Y, Kuo YF, et al. Potentially inappropriate screening colonoscopy in Medicare patients: variation by physician and geographic region. JAMA Intern Med 2013;173(7):542–50.
58. O'Brien MJ, Winawer SJ, Zauber AG, et al. The National Polyp Study. Patient and polyp characteristics associated with high-grade dysplasia in colorectal adenomas. Gastroenterology 1990;98(2):371–9.
59. SEER cancer statistics review 1973-1990. Bethesda, MD: US Department of Health and Human Services, Public Health Service, National Institutes of Health, National Cancer Institute; 1993.
60. Duncan JE, Sweeney WB, Trudel JL, et al. Colonoscopy in the elderly: low risk, low yield in asymptomatic patients. Dis Colon Rectum 2006;49(5):646–51.
61. Canada RE, Turner B. Talking to patients about screening colonoscopy—where conversations fall short. J Fam Pract 2007;56(8):E1–9.
62. Clarfield AM. Screening in frail older people: an ounce of prevention or a pound of trouble? J Am Geriatr Soc 2010;58(10):2016–21.
63. Torke AM, Schwartz PH, Holtz LR, et al. Older adults and forgoing cancer screening: "I think it would be strange." JAMA Intern Med 2013;173(7):526–31.
64. Warren JL, Klabunde CN, Mariotto AB, et al. Adverse events after outpatient colonoscopy in the Medicare population. Ann Intern Med 2009;150(12):849–57 W152.
65. Sheridan SL, Harris RP, Woolf SH. Shared decision making about screening and chemoprevention. A suggested approach from the U.S. Preventive Services Task Force. Am J Prev Med 2004;26(1):56–66.
66. Lewis CL, Golin CE, DeLeon C, et al. A targeted decision aid for the elderly to decide whether to undergo colorectal cancer screening: development and results of an uncontrolled trial. BMC Med Inform Decis Mak 2010;10:54.

67. Siegel JH, Kasmin FE. Biliary tract diseases in the elderly: management and outcomes. Gut 1997;41(4):433–5.
68. Katsinelos P, Kountouras J, Chatzimavroudis G, et al. Outpatient therapeutic endoscopic retrograde cholangiopancreatography is safe in patients aged 80 years and older. Endoscopy 2011;43(2):128–33.
69. Fritz E, Kirchgatterer A, Hubner D, et al. ERCP is safe and effective in patients 80 years of age and older compared with younger patients. Gastrointest Endosc 2006;64(6):899–905.
70. Katsinelos P, Paroutoglou G, Kountouras J, et al. Efficacy and safety of therapeutic ERCP in patients 90 years of age and older. Gastrointest Endosc 2006; 63(3):417–23.
71. Riphaus A, Stergiou N, Wehrmann T. ERCP in octogenerians: a safe and efficient investigation. Age Ageing 2008;37(5):595–9.
72. Loperfido S, Angelini G, Benedetti G, et al. Major early complications from diagnostic and therapeutic ERCP: a prospective multicenter study. Gastrointest Endosc 1998;48(1):1–10.
73. Mohammad Alizadeh AH, Afzali ES, Shahnazi A, et al. Utility and safety of ERCP in the elderly: a comparative study in Iran. Diagn Ther Endosc 2012;2012: 439320.
74. Laugier R, Bernard JP, Berthezene P, et al. Changes in pancreatic exocrine secretion with age: pancreatic exocrine secretion does decrease in the elderly. Digestion 1991;50(3–4):202–11.
75. Jenssen C, Alvarez-Sánchez MV, Napoléon B, et al. Diagnostic endoscopic ultrasonography: assessment of safety and prevention of complications. World J Gastroenterol 2012;18(34):4659–76.
76. Benson ME, Byrne S, Brust DJ, et al. EUS and ERCP complication rates are not increased in elderly patients. Dig Dis Sci 2010;55(11):3278–83.
77. Attila T, Faigel DO. Endoscopic ultrasound in patients over 80 years old. Dig Dis Sci 2011;56(10):3065–71.
78. Iles-Shih L, Hilden K, Adler DG. Combined ERCP and EUS in one session is safe in elderly patients when compared to non-elderly patients: outcomes in 206 combined procedures. Dig Dis Sci 2012;57(7):1949–53.
79. Potack JZ, Chokhavatia S. Complications of and controversies associated with percutaneous endoscopic gastrostomy: report of a case and literature review. Medscape J Med 2008;10(6):142.
80. Mendiratta P, Tilford JM, Prodhan P, et al. Trends in percutaneous endoscopic gastrostomy placement in the elderly from 1993 to 2003. Am J Alzheimers Dis Other Demen 2012;27(8):609–13.
81. Callahan CM, Haag KM, Weinberger M, et al. Outcomes of percutaneous endoscopic gastrostomy among older adults in a community setting. J Am Geriatr Soc 2000;48(9):1048–54.
82. Teno JM, Mitchell SL, Gozalo PL, et al. Hospital characteristics associated with feeding tube placement in nursing home residents with advanced cognitive impairment. JAMA 2010;303(6):544–50.
83. Sampson EL, Candy B, Jones L. Enteral tube feeding for older people with advanced dementia. Cochrane Database Syst Rev 2009;(2):CD007209.
84. Smoliner C, Volkert D, Wittrich A, et al. Basic geriatric assessment does not predict in-hospital mortality after PEG placement. BMC Geriatr 2012;12:52.
85. Kirby DF, Delegge MH, Fleming CR. American Gastroenterological Association technical review on tube feeding for enteral nutrition. Gastroenterology 1995; 108(4):1282–301.

86. Fisher L, Lee Krinsky M, Anderson MA, et al. The role of endoscopy in the management of obscure GI bleeding. Gastrointest Endosc 2010;72(3):471–9.
87. Ginsberg GG, Barkun AN, Bosco JJ, et al. Wireless capsule endoscopy August 2002. Gastrointest Endosc 2002;56(5):621–4.
88. Tsibouris P, Kalantzis C, Apostolopoulos P, et al. Capsule endoscopy findings in patients with occult or overt bleeding older than 80 years. Dig Endosc 2012; 24(3):154–8.
89. Gómez V, Cheesman AR, Heckman MG, et al. Safety of capsule endoscopy in the octogenarian as compared with younger patients. Gastrointest Endosc 2013;78(5):744–9.
90. Möschler O, May A, Müller MK, et al. Complications in and performance of double-balloon enteroscopy (DBE): results from a large prospective DBE database in Germany. Endoscopy 2011;43(6):484–9.
91. Sidhu R, Sanders DS. Double-balloon enteroscopy in the elderly with obscure gastrointestinal bleeding: safety and feasibility. Eur J Gastroenterol Hepatol 2013;25:1230–4.
92. Hegde SR, Iffrig K, Li T, et al. Double-balloon enteroscopy in the elderly: safety, findings, and diagnostic and therapeutic success. Gastrointest Endosc 2010; 71(6):983–9.

Hepatitis B and C

Anupama T. Duddempudi, MD[a],*, David E. Bernstein, MD[b]

KEYWORDS

- Hepatitis B • Hepatitis C • Elderly • Antiviral therapy • Interferon

KEY POINTS

- Hepatitis B and hepatitis C are common infections, which can lead to chronic liver disease, cirrhosis, and hepatocellular cancer; end-stage disease can be treated with liver transplantation.
- Significant progress in the evaluation and treatment of both diseases has been made in the past 20 years. Hepatitis B, although not curable, is suppressible with antiviral therapy, which has been shown to decrease liver disease morbidity and mortality.
- Elderly patients should be evaluated and treated for hepatitis in the same fashion as younger patients.
- Hepatitis C remains a major public health concern. Recent recommendations for birth cohort screening of all people in the United States born between 1945 and 1965 will increase the number of patients diagnosed with hepatitis C, especially among the elderly.
- A better understanding of the natural history of hepatitis C is needed. New methods of staging the disease will allow for noninvasive determination of fibrosis and allow more people to be adequately assessed for the disease.
- Newer, more efficacious therapies with fewer side effects and shorter durations of therapy should allow for more patients with hepatitis C to be treated, including the elderly, who remain an understudied and undertreated difficult-to-treat population with hepatitis C infection.

HEPATITIS B
Introduction

Hepatitis B virus (HBV) is a double-stranded DNA virus belonging to the family of hepadnaviruses and is classified into 8 genotypes (A–H). The prevalence of specific genotypes varies geographically. Perinatal and horizontal transmission early in life are most common in high-prevalence areas such as Southeast Asia and China, whereas sexual contact and percutaneous transmission (eg, intravenous drug use) are most common in the United States, Canada, and Western Europe.

[a] Division of Hepatology, North Shore University Hospital, Hofstra North Shore LIJ School of Medicine, 300 Community Drive, Manhasset, NY 11030, USA; [b] Division of Hepatology and Center for Liver Disease, North Shore Long Island Jewish Health System, Hofstra North Shore LIJ School of Medicine, 300 Community Drive, Manhasset, NY 11030, USA
* Corresponding author.
E-mail address: aduddempudi@nshs.edu

Clin Geriatr Med 30 (2014) 149–167
http://dx.doi.org/10.1016/j.cger.2013.10.012   geriatric.theclinics.com
0749-0690/14/$ – see front matter © 2014 Elsevier Inc. All rights reserved.

HBV infection is a global public health problem. It is estimated that there are more than 350 million HBV carriers in the world,[1] of whom approximately 500,000 die annually from HBV-related liver disease.

Serologic Assays

The diagnosis of HBV was revolutionized by the discovery of the Australia antigen now called hepatitis B surface antigen (HBsAg) more than 4 decades ago. Since then, serologic assays have been established for HBV antigens and antibodies as well as polymerase chain reaction (PCR) assays for determination of viral load. HBV DNA viral testing is used to assess HBV replication and determine the indication for and response to antiviral therapy.

HBsAg is the serologic hallmark for infection. In the case of an acute exposure to HBV, the antigen is detectable 1 to 10 weeks after exposure, before any symptoms or increase in alanine transaminase (ALT) levels. When the antigen has been present for more than 6 months, the patient has a chronic infection.

The anti–hepatitis B core antibody (anti-HBc) assay is used to detect antibodies to the hepatitis B core antigen, an intracellular antigen expressed in infected hepatocytes that cannot be detected in serum. During acute infection, the anti-HBc is mainly IgM class and can be detectable for up to 2 years after the infection. After resolution of acute infection or progression to chronic infection, the anti-HBc is mainly IgG class.

The hepatitis B e antigen (HBeAg) is a marker of HBV replication and infectivity and is associated with high levels of DNA in serum and higher rates of disease transmission. Conversion of HBeAg to anti–hepatitis B e antibody (anti-HBe) occurs early during acute infection but later in chronic infection. HbeAg-positive patients with infection acquired perinatally can have a normal ALT level and minimal inflammation in the liver.[1,2] Seroconversion from HBeAg to anti-HBe usually leads to decreased HBV DNA levels as well as remission of activity at the hepatocyte level.[3,4]

Serologic markers are used to determine the clinical phase of an acute or chronic infection as well as identify patients in need of immunization (**Table 1**).

Screening

Risk factors for HBV have been determined and should be used to identify patients with possible hepatitis B infection (**Box 1**).[1] Initial testing should include HBsAg, anti-HBc, and anti-HBs. Patients who are negative for these markers should be vaccinated. HBsAg-positive pregnant women should inform their providers so that their infants can receive hepatitis B immune globulin and vaccine immediately after delivery.

Carriers of HBV should be counseled regarding the risk of transmission to others and have a complete evaluation, including evaluation for other causes of liver disease and screening for hepatocellular carcinoma (HCC).

Acute Hepatitis B

Acute hepatitis B manifestations range from subclinical hepatitis in approximately 70% of patients to icteric hepatitis in 30% and fulminant hepatitis in 0.1% to 0.5% of patients. The incubation period is 1 to 4 months. Patients may develop a serum sicknesslike syndrome during the prodromal period followed by anorexia, nausea, jaundice, and right upper quadrant pain. The symptoms usually resolve within 3 months, but some patients have prolonged fatigue. Laboratory testing during this period shows increased aspartate transaminase and ALT levels, with possible increase of bilirubin levels as well. The prothrombin time is the best indicator of prognosis.

Table 1
Hepatitis B serologic panel interpretation

Tests	Results	Interpretation
HBsAg Anti-HBc Anti-HBs	Negative Negative Negative	Susceptible and should be immunized
HBsAg Anti-HBc Anti-HBs	Negative Positive Positive	Immune because of previous exposure
HBsAg Anti-HBc Anti-HBs	Negative Negative Positive	Immune because of vaccination
HBsAg Anti-HBc Anti-HBs IgM anti-HBc	Positive Positive Negative Positive	Acute or reactivation infection
HBsAg Anti-HBc Anti-HBs IgM anti-HBc	Positive Positive or negative Positive or negative Negative	Chronic infection
HBsAg Anti-HBc Anti-HBs	Negative Positive Negative	False positive anti-HBc, distantly immune, recovery phase of acute infection or very low levels of HBsAg which would mean chronic infection

The rate of progression from acute to chronic disease is determined by initial age at infection. For perinatal infections, the rate to development of chronic hepatitis B is 90%, 20% to 50% for age 1 to 5 years, and less than 5% for adult acquired infection.[5]

Treatment of acute hepatitis B is mainly supportive and should include appropriate measures to prevent infection in exposed contacts. Patients with coagulopathy, jaundice, or encephalopathy should be considered for more intensive follow-up, which may include hospitalization or the initiation of antiviral therapy. Older patients, those with significant comorbidities, or those who cannot tolerate oral intake should be hospitalized.

The overall recommendation for supportive care rather than treatment with antiviral therapy has been supported by Kumar and colleagues,[6] who showed that patients

Box 1
Risk factors for hepatitis B

People born in Asia, Africa, Middle East, South Pacific Islands, South America, Eastern Europe, Mediterranean

US-born persons not vaccinated as infants whose parents were born in high-risk regions

Household and sexual contacts of HBsAg-positive persons

Men who have sex with men

Intravenous drug use

Multiple sexual partners

Inmates of correctional facilities

Renal dialysis

receiving lamivudine for acute hepatitis B had no biochemical or clinical benefit compared with the placebo group. However, the role of antiviral therapy in patients with severe or protracted acute infection was not adequately addressed nor was the current standard of care therapies for chronic hepatitis B evaluated.

Current recommendations from the American Association for the Study of Liver Disease (AASLD) are to treat patients with acute hepatitis B with antiviral therapy if a severe or protracted course is present for more than 4 weeks or if the patient is immunocompromised, elderly, or has preexisting liver disease.[1] Telbivudine, lamivudine, tenofovir, or entecavir are all acceptable options, given as monotherapy, because the duration of treatment should be short. Treatment can be stopped after confirmation (2 consecutive tests 4 weeks apart) that the patient has cleared HBsAg. Interferon should be avoided in the acute setting, because of the risk of exacerbating the acute inflammatory response as a result of the possible ALT flare seen with interferon therapy.

Chronic Hepatitis B

Most patients with chronic hepatitis B are asymptomatic unless they have decompensated cirrhosis or extrahepatic manifestations. In decompensated cirrhosis, jaundice, coagulopathy, ascites, and encephalopathy can be present. Extrahepatic manifestations occur in about 10% to 20% of chronic infections and are believed to be mediated by circulating immune complexes. The 2 major complications seen are polyarteritis nodosa, which responds to antiviral therapy, and glomerular disease, which mainly occurs in children.

Phases of infection

Chronic HBV infection generally consists of 2 phases: an early replicative phase, with active liver disease, and a later phase, with low replication and remission of liver disease.[1,3,4] In patients with perinatally acquired HBV infection, there is an additional immune tolerance phase, in which virus replication is not accompanied by active liver disease.[7]

Replicative phase: immune tolerance In patients with perinatally acquired HBV infection, the initial phase is characterized by high levels of HBV replication but no evidence of active liver disease, with normal serum ALT concentrations and minimal changes on liver biopsy.[1,2] One study also showed that fibrosis scores on repeat biopsies were unchanged after 5 years among patients who remained in the immune-tolerant phase.[8] The lack of liver disease despite high levels of HBV replication is believed to be caused by immune tolerance to HBV, but the mechanism is unknown.[9] This is also believed to be the major reason for the poor response to interferon therapy in HBeAg-positive Asian patients who have normal serum ALT concentrations.

This phase can last up to 30 years, during which there is a very low rate of spontaneous HBeAg clearance.[10,11] The cumulative rate of spontaneous HBeAg clearance is approximately 2% during the first 3 years and 15% after 20 years of infection.[11]

Replicative phase: immune clearance During the immune clearance phase, spontaneous HBeAg clearance increases to 10% to 20% per year. Several studies from Asia have found that patients with genotype B infection undergo HBeAg seroconversion at an earlier age than those with genotype C infection.[10,11]

HBeAg seroconversion is frequently accompanied by increases in ALT levels and an increase in serum HBV DNA, but generally, patients remain asymptomatic. For unclear reasons, reactivation is more commonly observed in men more than in women.[12,13] Patients with severe reactivation should be referred to specialized centers for liver transplantation or oral antiviral treatment. Interferon should be avoided in this scenario, because it can worsen the disease state.

Some patients, despite reactivation, do not have seroconversion and clearance of HBV DNA from the serum and remain with chronic disease. Multiple reactivations is associated with an increased risk of developing cirrhosis and HCC.

Low or nonreplication phase/inactive carrier state Previously termed healthy carriers, these patients are characterized by a pattern of being HBeAg negative and anti-HBe positive, with low HBV viral loads and liver disease that is in remission. However, studies have shown that significant liver disease can be found in patients with HBeAg-negative chronic HBV, but this is rare in those with persistently normal ALT levels and HBV DNA levels less than 2000 IU/mL.[14–16] For these reasons, the terminology of healthy carrier should be abandoned.

Because of the fluctuating nature of chronic HBV infection, patients should not be categorized as inactive carriers unless they have at least 3 ALT levels and 2 to 3 HBV DNA levels that meet the criteria listed earlier over a 12-month period of observation.

Some patients who are HBeAg negative can have moderate levels of HBV replication and active liver disease and are believed to have a residual wild-type virus or HBV variants that cannot produce HBeAg because of precore or core promoter genetic variations.[17,18] These patients tend to be older and have more advanced liver disease.

Resolution of chronic HBV infection
The annual rate of delayed clearance of HBsAg is 0.5% to 2% in Western countries compared with 0.1% to 0.8% in Asian countries.[19,20] Despite a generally favorable prognosis, clearance of HBsAg does not preclude the development of cirrhosis or HCC.[21,22] In 1 report, the likelihood of developing HCC was greater in those who cleared HBsAg when older than 50 years.[23] Furthermore, some of the patients may have had undocumented cirrhosis or irreversible liver damage before seroconversion.

Many patients who clear HBsAg remain HBV DNA positive when tested by PCR assays, particularly during the first 10 years after HBsAg clearance.[23] A reactivation of HBV replication with reappearance of HBeAg and HBV DNA (by hybridization assays) in serum and recrudescence of liver disease may occur when these patients are immunosuppressed or receive systemic cancer chemotherapy, systemic corticosteroids, or biological agents. The disease reactivation can vary in severity from mild and asymptomatic to severe with possible fulminant hepatic failure, resulting in the need for liver transplantation or death.

Prognosis with chronic infection
The estimated 5-year rates of progression from chronic hepatitis to cirrhosis is 12% to 20%; compensated cirrhosis to hepatic decompensation, 20% to 23%; and compensated cirrhosis to HCC, 6% to 15%.[24] The risk of progression seems to be greatest in patients who remain in the immune clearance phase, in patients who have delayed HBeAg seroconversion, and in patients who have had a reactivation of HBV replication after HBeAg seroconversion.[25,26]

However, these rates of progression were based on data in the preoral antiviral treatment era, and these treatments have changed the disease course in many treated patients.

HBV DNA levels correlate with progression to cirrhosis, as seen in the REVEAL HBV (Risk Evaluation of Viral Load Elevation and Associated Liver Disease/Cancer–Hepatitis B Virus) study,[27] which reported that over an 11-year period, the incidence of cirrhosis in patients with a viral load less than 300 copies/mL was 4.5% compared with 36% in patients with viral load greater than 10^6 copies/mL. The HBV DNA level remained an independent predictor of the development of cirrhosis after adjusting for HBeAg status, age, sex, ALT level, cigarette smoking, and alcohol consumption. High serum HBV DNA ($>10^6$ copies/mL) was also an independent predictor of the development of HCC.[28]

In patients with HbeAg-negative chronic HBV with a low HBV viral load, HBsAg levels greater than 1000 UI/mL have been associated with an increased risk of disease progression and the development of HCC.[29]

Confection with Hepatitis C Virus or Hepatitis D Virus

Coexistent hepatitis C virus (HCV) infection has been estimated to be present in 10% to 15% of patients with HBV.[30] HCV superinfection in HBsAg carriers seems to reduce HBV DNA levels and increase the rate of HBsAg seroconversion.[31,32] Most patients with HBV/HCV coinfection have detectable serum HCV RNA but undetectable or low HBV DNA levels, indicating that HCV is the predominant cause of liver disease in these patients. Liver disease is usually more severe than in patients infected by HBV alone.[33]

For hepatitis D virus (HDV) infection, the presence of HBV is required for the HDV to replicate. HDV is endemic, particularly in Eastern Europe, Mediterranean countries, and the Amazon basin. It is uncommon in the United States. Acute HBV and HDV co-infection tends to be more severe than acute HBV infection alone and is more likely to result in fulminant hepatitis.[34] HDV superinfection in patients with chronic HBV infection is usually accompanied by a suppression of HBV replication, which is not well understood.[35] HDV superinfection has been associated with more advanced liver disease and accelerated progression to cirrhosis.[36,37]

Treatment of HBV

Given the risk of progressive liver disease, patients who meet the criteria should be considered for treatment.

Patients with compensated cirrhosis and HBV DNA levels of greater than 2000 IU/mL and those with decompensated cirrhosis and detectable HBV DNA by PCR assay should be considered for antiviral therapy, regardless of the serum ALT level.

AASLD recommendations for the treatment of chronic hepatitis C are shown in **Fig. 1**.[1] Recommendations from the European Association for the Study of the Liver, which were updated in 2012, suggest that patients be considered for treatment when they have HBV DNA levels greater than 2000 IU/mL, have serum ALT levels higher than the upper limit of normal, and have evidence of moderate to severe necroinflammation or at least moderate fibrosis on liver biopsy (or assessed using a validated noninvasive marker).[38]

HBeAg-positive patients

Treatment is recommended for those patients with HBV DNA levels greater than 20,000 IU/mL and ALT levels greater than 2 times the upper limit of normal in patients without cirrhosis. Treatment should be delayed for 3 to 6 months in newly diagnosed HbeAg-positive patients with compensated liver disease to determine whether spontaneous HBeAg seroconversion will occur. However, if the patient has recurrent hepatitis flares that fail to clear HBeAg, or active or advanced histologic findings or is older than 40 years, treatment should be considered.[1]

HBeAg-negative patients

Treatment is recommended for patients whose ALT is greater than 2 times the upper limit of normal and HBV DNA levels are greater than 2000 IU/mL. Liver biopsy should

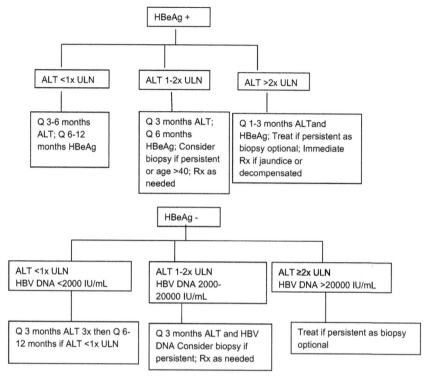

Fig. 1. Management of HBV (AASLD guidelines).

be considered in HbeAg-negative patients who have serum HBV DNA levels of greater than 2000 IU/mL and normal or mildly increased ALT levels to determine if treatment is warranted.

Treatment options

Interferon Interferon α, an injectable medication, may be administered at a dose of 5 million units daily, 10 million units 3 times a week, or as a once-weekly injection for a duration of 16 to 24 weeks in HbeAg- positive patients and at least 12 months in HbeAg-negative patients. Interferon therapy results in a 60% to 70% loss of HBV DNA, 60% to 70% normalization of ALT levels, and a 10% to 20% durability of response.[1] Pegylated interferon is associated with a 48% improvement in liver histology.[1] The advantage of interferon is the finite duration of treatment compared with other treatments. There is also the absence of selection of resistant mutants and a more durable response. There are several disadvantages to interferon use. The side effects of interferon are significant for many patients, especially the elderly, and the need for multiple injections compared with other all-oral therapies may lead to less patient acceptance of this therapy. Furthermore, interferon cannot be used in patients with cirrhosis, decompensated disease, or active or reactivation disease.

Lamivudine Lamivudine was the first oral agent approved for use in chronic hepatitis B infection. Lamivudine therapy results in a 60% to 73% loss of HBV DNA, 60% to 79% normalization of ALT levels, 60% to 66% improvement in liver histology, and a less than 10% durability of response.[1] Its main advantages are low cost and the many years of experience confirming its safety, including its use during pregnancy. However, there is a high rate of drug resistance, 70% at 4 years, which severely limits its long-term use.[38] The role of lamivudine in the care of HBV is diminishing with the availability of new therapies, which are associated with lower rates of drug resistance.

Adefovir Adefovir was mainly used for lamivudine-resistant HBV, because it has a lower rate of drug resistance compared with lamivudine. Adefovir therapy results in a 51% loss of HBV DNA, 72% normalization of ALT levels, 64% improvement in liver histology, and a less than 5% durability of response.[1] At high doses, adefovir has been associated with nephrotoxicity. The rate of drug resistance has been reported to be as high as 29% after 5 years of treatment.[38]

Telbivudine Telbivudine therapy results in an 88% loss of HBV DNA, 74% normalization of ALT levels, and a 67% improvement in liver histology.[1] Telbivudine has a high rate of resistant mutation development at 2 years therapy (17%).[38] Its role as primary therapy is limited. Myopathy has been reported with telbivudine use.[38]

Entecavir Entecavir therapy results in a 90% loss of HBV DNA, 78% normalization of ALT levels, and 70% improvement in liver histology.[1] The main advantages of entecavir are its potent antiviral activity and a low rate of drug resistance (<1%).[1]

Tenofovir Tenofovir therapy results in a 93% loss of HBV DNA, 76% normalization of ALT levels, and 72% improvement in liver histology.[1] The main advantages of tenofovir are its potent antiviral effects and lack of reported drug resistance.[38]

Treatment End Points

The optimal duration of therapy for the oral drugs is not well established. Most patients require at least 4 to 5 years of treatment, and some may require indefinite treatment. In patients who are HBeAg positive, the end point after 1 year is HBeAg seroconversion and undetectable HBV DNA. If therapy is discontinued, patients should be closely monitored after discontinuation of treatment of viral relapse. In patients who are HBeAg negative, there is no defined end point. Treatment may be discontinued in patients who have confirmed loss of HBsAg and HBsAb seroconversion, but this is uncommon, occurring in less than 5% of patients after 5 years of continued therapy.[1,38]

In patients with compensated cirrhosis, lifelong treatment is recommended to prevent HCC and decompensation, but discontinuing treatment can be considered if the patient has a hepatitis B surface antibody seroconversion.[1,38] For decompensated cirrhosis, lifelong treatment is recommended.[1,38]

Hepatitis B in the Elderly: Special Considerations

The prevalence of hepatitis B among people older than 50 years in the United States is significantly greater than in those younger than 50 years.[39] Clinical manifestations of chronic hepatitis B in the elderly are similar to those of a younger population, but the manifestations of acute disease differ with more presentations of asymptomatic acute disease and fewer episodes of jaundice and fulminant disease. Patients acutely infected with hepatitis B older than 65 years are less likely to clear infection and more likely to develop chronic disease, at a rate of 59%.[40] Chronically infected individuals aged 60 years or older are more likely to spontaneously clear HBsAg than younger patients.[20] Adults older than 60 years are 4 times more likely to be HBeAg positive than those younger than 40 years.[41]

Treatment of hepatitis B is not dependent on age, and the elderly should be treated if appropriate treatment criteria are met. Interferon, with its side effect profile, may best be avoided in the elderly. Entecavir and tenofovir, which are the recommended agents of choice for the treatment of chronic hepatitis B,[1,38] should be used with caution in the elderly. These agents are excreted by the kidney and must be dose reduced for a creatinine clearance less than 50. Elderly patients on these therapies should have their creatinine clearance and serum phosphate levels monitored during therapy at initial intervals of every 3 months for 1 year and then every 6 months for the duration of therapy.[38]

Elderly patients receiving chemotherapy, systemic corticosteroids, biological response modifiers, and other forms of immunosuppression should be checked for the presence of hepatitis B before initiation of these therapies, because these agents may be associated with disease reactivation. **Screening for hepatitis B in this population should include HBsAg and anti-HBc, and those who are positive should be tested for the presence of HBV DNA**. Certain patients may require prophylaxis before initiation of these therapies. If prophylaxis is required, current recommendations are for lamivudine or telbivudine if the anticipated duration is less than 12 months and tenofovir or entecavir if longer treatment is anticipated.[1,38]

Nursing home residents have an increased risk of hepatitis B acquisition, and the prevalence of hepatitis B infection has been found to be higher in nursing home residents than in noninstitutionalized residents of similar age.[42] Because of this situation, it is recommended that all nursing home residents and their health care providers be vaccinated against hepatitis B.

HEPATITIS C
Introduction

HCV can cause both acute and chronic hepatitis. The acute process is self-limited, rarely causes hepatic failure, and leads to chronic infection in 60% to 80% patients. Chronic HCV infection often follows a progressive course over many years and can result in cirrhosis, HCC, and the need for liver transplantation. In the United States, chronic HCV is the most common cause of chronic viral liver disease and the most frequent indication for liver transplantation.[43]

Because of the long course of the disease, it is difficult to define the natural history. A review of 111 studies evaluating the natural history estimated that the prevalence of cirrhosis was 16% after 20 years.[44] However, not all patients have progressive disease, and mortality is not always related to liver disease. Cirrhosis occurs in about half the chronically infected patients.[45,46] Once advanced fibrosis has occurred, the risk of progressing to cirrhosis is 10% a year. The risk of decompensation is approximately 3.9% a year.[47]

The hallmark of decompensated disease is the appearance of ascites, variceal bleeding, encephalopathy jaundice, or HCC. Hepatitis C also accounts for a third of the HCC cases in the United States. However, deaths associated with HCV in the United States are more likely caused by end-stage liver disease than HCC.[47] The risk of developing HCC is estimated to be approximately 3% a year.[47] It also seems to be greater in patients with genotype 1b than in those with genotype 2a/c.[48]

The reason for the differences in susceptibility among individual patients is not clear, but host and viral factors may play a role. Host factors that have been studied include high BMI, hepatic steatosis, insulin resistance, alcohol intake, and marijuana use. The effect of viral factors such as viral load and genotype on progression is less certain.

Screening for Hepatitis C

Screening for hepatitis C is initially performed through serologic assays that detect antibodies to hepatitis C, followed by confirmatory molecular assays that detect and quantify HCV RNA in those patients with positive hepatitis C antibody. Historically, patients chosen for hepatitis C testing were those found to have increased liver enzyme levels or those who had 1 or more risk factors for the disease (**Box 2**). However, in August, 2012, the US Centers for Disease Control (CDC) recommended that all people born between 1945 and 1965 be tested once for hepatitis C, including those without identifiable HCV risk factors.[49] The United States Preventative Services Task Force endorsed this recommendation in 2013.[50]

Management of Hepatitis C

Management focuses not only on antiviral therapy but also on psychological counseling and symptom management, as well as screening for complications of cirrhosis. Because of common modes of transmission, patients should be screened for HIV and hepatitis B as well. In addition, patients should be tested for hepatitis A to determine if vaccination is required to prevent the acquisition of hepatitis A or B.

Counseling

Although most patients are asymptomatic, the diagnosis can have important emotional and physical consequences. Patients should be offered counseling and screening for depression, and may benefit from participation in a support group. Education should be provided about the routes of HCV transmission as well as factors that promote hepatic fibrosis, such as alcohol and obesity.

Symptom management

Many patients with HCV who are otherwise asymptomatic complain of fatigue even before the diagnosis. The cause of the fatigue is uncertain and may improve after hepatitis C treatment. One large study of 431 patients who underwent treatment of HCV reported that fatigue improved significantly more often in responders than in nonresponders (35 vs 22%) to antiviral therapy.[51] Ondansetron (a 5-HT3 receptor antagonist) was found to significantly improve fatigue in a placebo-controlled trial of 36 patients.[52] Long-term efficacy of ondansetron is unclear, and adverse effects include constipation and cardiac arrhythmias.

Patients can also present with extrahepatic manifestations of chronic hepatitis C, which seem to be directly related to the viral infection. In 1 study of 321 patients,

---

Box 2
Risk factors for hepatitis C

Illicit injection drug use

Intranasal cocaine use

Received clotting factors made before 1987

Receiving a blood transfusion or organ transplant before July, 1992

Long-term hemodialysis

Needlestick exposure

Children born to hepatitis C virus–positive mothers

Human immunodeficiency virus coinfection

History of incarceration

Sexual partner with hepatitis C virus

Unregulated tattoo

38% patients had at least 1 extrahepatic manifestation (**Table 2**).[53] Certain extrahepatic manifestations, such as cryoglobulinemia, porphyria cutanea tarda, leukocytoclastic vasculitis, necrolytic acral erythema, and glomerulonephritis, respond to HCV treatment.

Cirrhosis can lead to esophageal variceal bleeding as well as HCC. Patients with cirrhosis should be screened for the presence of esophageal varices with upper endoscopy and undergo surveillance for HCC with imaging twice a year.

Antiviral Therapy

The goal of therapy is to eradicate HCV RNA and have a sustained virologic response (SVR). SVR is associated with a 97% to 100% chance of being HCV RNA negative during long-term follow-up and has been associated with a decrease in all-cause mortality, liver-related death, the need for liver transplantation, HCC, and liver-related complications, even in those patients with advanced liver fibrosis.[54–57]

Patients must be carefully selected for current HCV therapy. The decision to treat is based on multiple factors, including genotype, fibrosis stage, patient motivation, and the efficacy and adverse effects related to therapy. Genotype testing helps determine the choice of therapy and the duration of therapy and predicts the likelihood of obtaining an SVR.

Table 2	
Extrahepatic manifestations of HCV infection	
Skin	**%**
Purpura	7
Raynaud phenomenon	7
Cutaneous vasculitis	6
Pruritus	6
Psoriasis	20
Porphyria cutanea tarda	1
Lichen planus	1
At least 1 skin manifestation	17
Rheumatologic	
Arthralgia	19
Arthritis	2
Myalgia	2
Neurologic	
Sensory neuropathy	9
Motor neuropathy	5
Miscellaneous	
Sicca syndrome (eye)	10
Sicca syndrome (mouth)	12
Hypertension	10
Uveitis	1
At least 1 extrahepatic clinical manifestation	38

Data from Cacoub P, Renou C, Rosenthal E, et al. Extrahepatic manifestations associated with hepatitis C virus infection. A prospective multicenter study of 321 patients. The GERMIVIC. Groupe d'Etude et de Recherche en Medecine Interne et Maladies Infectieuses sur le Virus de l'Hepatitis C. Medicine (Baltimore) 2000;79:47.

Fibrosis

Hepatic fibrosis occurs in response to chronic liver injury, regardless of the cause. It is a dynamic process, with potential for reversal and resolution. Determining fibrosis is critical in the management of patients with hepatitis C. Patients with advanced fibrosis tend to have a lower response to treatment. Treatment may be delayed or deferred if minimal fibrosis is present.

Liver biopsy is considered to be the gold standard for the staging of hepatic fibrosis. Liver biopsy may also help exclude other liver diseases, such as autoimmune hepatitis or iron overload.

In recent years, noninvasive serologic tests and transient elastography have been developed as an alternative to liver biopsy to assess hepatic fibrosis. Serologic testing is more readily available, because transient elastography has only recently been approved in the United States. Serologic tests can differentiate patients with significant fibrosis (F2–F4) from minimal fibrosis (F0–F1). Serologic testing does not reliably differentiate between moderate and severe fibrosis.[58]

Ultrasound-based transient elastography was approved for use in the United States in 2013. This technology measures liver stiffness using a section of liver that is approximately 1 cm by 5 cm, an area that is approximately 100 times larger than a liver biopsy and therefore more representative of the hepatic parenchyma.[58] A meta-analysis of 9 studies[59] showed that transient elastography had an 87% sensitivity and 91% specificity for diagnosing cirrhosis and a 70% sensitivity and 84% specificity for diagnosing significant fibrosis. Factors that reduce the accuracy of transient elastography include ascites, increased central venous pressure (heart failure), and obesity.

In the future, it may be feasible to use a combination of tests, such as a serologic panel and transient elastography, to better assess underlying liver fibrosis in a highly accurate and noninvasive fashion and without needing a liver biopsy to garner this important clinical information.

Treatment options

The current standard of care is to treat patients with genotype 1 with pegylated interferon, ribavirin, and a protease inhibitor, either telaprevir or boceprevir, which are considered direct-acting antiviral therapy. Patients with other genotypes are currently treated with pegylated interferon and ribavirin.[43] Treatment is generally indicated in patients with a detectable viral load, fibrosis, and without contraindications to treatment. Changes in viral load during therapy are used to determine if a patient is responding to treatment and to predict whether the patient is likely to eradicate the virus. The earlier the HCV RNA becomes undetectable during treatment, the more likely a patient is to eradicate the virus and develop an SVR. Response-guided therapy, in which the length of treatment is determined by virologic response, has become the standard method of determining treatment duration.[60] Patients with cirrhosis are not eligible for response-guided therapy and are treated for 48 weeks with telaprevir-based or boceprevir-based regimens.[60]

For patients with genotype 1, protease inhibitor–based therapy leads to SVR rates of 70% to 80%.[61] Patients with genotype 2 and 3 treated with pegylated interferon and ribavirin have SVR rates of 70% to 80%.[61]

Contraindications for interferon-based therapy include active major depression, autoimmune disorders, and pregnancy. A more comprehensive list of adverse events is listed in **Table 3**.[60]

Patients receiving telaprevir or boceprevir are at increased risk for developing anemia. Telaprevir is frequently associated with rashes.[60] Care of patients with chronic hepatitis C depends on recognition of those at increased risk for side effects,

Table 3 Adverse effects of peginterferon, ribavirin, and protease inhibitors	
Medication	**Side Effect**
Peginterferon	Flulike symptoms
	Anemia
	Neutropenia
	Thrombocytopenia
	Rashes
	Hair loss
	Thyroid dysfunction
	Depression
	Fatigue
	Irritability and mania
	Nonproductive cough
	Dyspnea
	Ophthalmologic disorders such as retinal hemorrhages
	Teratogenicity
	Exacerbations of autoimmune diseases
Ribavirin	Hemolytic anemia
	Rash
	Nonproductive cough
Telaprevir	Rash
	Pruritus
	Anemia
	Nausea
	Hemorrhoids
	Anorectal discomfort
	Diarrhea
	Dysgeusia
	Fatigue
	Vomiting
	Anal pruritus
Boceprevir	Fatigue
	Anemia
	Nausea
	Headache
	Dysgeusia
	Dry mouth
	Vomiting
	Diarrhea

anticipation (and prevention) of side effects, and appropriate intervention when adverse events occur. The ability to achieve an SVR is dependent on the degree of compliance with therapy.[60]

Future Directions in Hepatitis C Therapy

The treatment of hepatitis C is undergoing a rapid change, with many new, potentially more efficacious, and better tolerated therapies on the horizon. Newer, all-oral therapies for genotype 2 and 3 are likely to be approved before newer all-oral regimens are available for genotypes 1, 4, and 5. Newer regimens for the treatment of genotypes 1, 4, and 5 combining pegylated interferon, ribavirin, and other classes of direct-acting antiviral therapies such as newer protease inhibitors, polymerase inhibitors, NS5A inhibitors, and NS5B inhibitors are likely to become available in the near future. These therapies seem to be more efficacious, better tolerated, and of shorter duration than currently available treatment options and offer hope that most patients with hepatitis C can be treated and cured.[62–65]

Hepatitis C in the Elderly: Special Considerations

Although the prevalence of hepatitis C is estimated to be about 3% of the global population,[66] the estimated prevalence of hepatitis C in the elderly population is significantly higher. Cainelli[67] estimated the prevalence of hepatitis C infection in individuals in Italy older than 60 years to be approximately 40%. Other prevalence studies[68–72] have described a prevalence of 1% to 11% in people older than 60 years. Risk factor specific screening yielded a prevalence of HCV infection of 87% in elderly individuals with a history of abnormal ALT levels or blood transfusions before 1992.[69] With the adoption of the CDC and US Services Preventive Task Force recommendation for cohort screening of all individuals born between 1945 and 1965, the number of elderly patients diagnosed with hepatitis C in the United States is likely to increase significantly. In addition to common risk factors for hepatitis C infection, older individuals are more likely to have received blood transfusions before 1992 or served in the military as a young adult, another potential risk factor for hepatitis C.

The natural history of hepatitis C in the elderly is unclear, although older individuals are more likely to present with more advanced disease, including cirrhosis and HCC.[73] Older, newly infected individuals progress more rapidly to advanced disease than younger newly infected individuals, with the mean time to cirrhosis described as 16 years in the older group compared with 33 years in the younger group.[74,75] Several investigators have concluded that the time to the development of cirrhosis and HCC in individuals who were infected with HCV after blood transfusions after the age of 50 years is more rapid than in younger patients.[45,76]

Elderly individuals with hepatitis C are more likely to have a normal ALT level than younger counterparts. Because the elderly population is less likely to undergo liver biopsy for disease staging, the value of using noninvasive markers of fibrosis and transient elastography, despite their shortcomings, becomes heightened.

Few studies have examined the treatment of older adults with hepatitis C. Most clinical treatment trials have excluded subjects older than 70 years. Elderly patients are less likely in clinical practice to be offered current antiviral therapy because of concerns regarding medication adverse events and comorbid illnesses, especially heart, pulmonary, and hematologic diseases and depression. These factors led the National Institutes of Health Consensus Conference to identify elderly patients as a difficult-to-treat group.[77] One small study of 33 patients suggested a lower SVR rate (46%) in elderly patients with a mean age of 70.2 years when compared with younger patients (69%) when treated with pegylated interferon and ribavirin.[78] No data are available to assess the efficacy and adverse event profile of the protease inhibitors telaprevir and boceprevir in the treatment of elderly patients. The hope for the treatment of elderly patients with chronic hepatitis C is that the new pipeline of medications, which are more efficacious, have fewer adverse events, have shorter treatment durations and are all oral, will allow this difficult-to-treat patient group to be safely treated.

SUMMARY

Hepatitis B and hepatitis C are common infections, which can lead to chronic liver disease, cirrhosis, hepatocellular cancer; end-stage disease can be treated with liver transplantation. Significant progress in the evaluation and treatment of both diseases has been made in the past 20 years. Hepatitis B, although not curable, is suppressible with antiviral therapy, which has been shown to decrease liver disease morbidity and mortality. Elderly patients should be evaluated and treated for hepatitis in the same fashion as those of younger ages.

Hepatitis C remains a major public health concern. Recent recommendations for birth cohort screening of all people in the United States born between 1945 and 1965 will increase the number of patients diagnosed with hepatitis C, especially among the elderly. A better understanding of the natural history of hepatitis C is needed. New methods of staging the disease will allow for noninvasive determination of fibrosis and allow more people to be adequately assessed for the disease. Newer, more efficacious therapies with fewer side effects and shorter durations of therapy should allow for more patients with hepatitis C to be treated, including the elderly, who remain an understudied and undertreated difficult-to-treat population with hepatitis C infection.

REFERENCES

1. Lok AS, McMahon BJ. Chronic hepatitis B. Hepatology 2009;50:1–36.
2. Chang MH, Hwang LY, Hsu HC, et al. Prospective study of asymptomatic HBsAg carrier children infected in the perinatal period: clinical and liver histologic studies. Hepatology 1988;8:374–7.
3. Hoofnagle JH, Dusheiko GM, Seeff LB, et al. Seroconversion from hepatitis B e antigen to antibody in chronic type B hepatitis. Ann Intern Med 1981;94:744–8.
4. Realdi G, Alberti A, Rugge M, et al. Seroconversion from hepatitis B e antigen to anti-HBe in chronic hepatitis B virus infection. Gastroenterology 1980;79:195–9.
5. Tassopoulous NC, Papaevangelou GJ, Sjogren MH, et al. Natural history of acute hepatitis B surface antigen-positive hepatitis in Greek adults. Gastroenterology 1987;92:1844–50.
6. Kumar M, Satapathy S, Monga R, et al. A randomized controlled trial of lamivudine to treat acute hepatitis B. Hepatology 2007;45:97–101.
7. Lok AS. Natural history and control of perinatally acquired hepatitis B virus infection. Dig Dis 1992;10:46–52.
8. Hui CK, Leung N, Yuen ST, et al. Natural history and disease progression in Chinese chronic hepatitis B patients in immune-tolerant phase. Hepatology 2007; 46:395–401.
9. Hsu HY, Chang MH, Hsieh KH, et al. Cellular immune response to HBcAg in mother-to-infant transmission of hepatitis B virus. Hepatology 1992;15:770–6.
10. Liaw YF, Chu CM, Lin DY, et al. Age-specific prevalence and significance of hepatitis B e antigen and antibody in chronic hepatitis B virus infection in Taiwan: a comparison among asymptomatic carriers, chronic hepatitis, liver cirrhosis and hepatocellular carcinoma. J Med Virol 1984;13:385–91.
11. Lok AS, Lai CL, Wu PC, et al. Spontaneous hepatitis B e antigen to antibody seroconversion and reversion in Chinese patients with chronic hepatitis B virus infection. Gastroenterology 1987;92:1839–43.
12. Kumar M, Chauhan R, Gupta N, et al. Spontaneous increases in alanine aminotransferase levels in asymptomatic chronic hepatitis B virus-infected patients. Gastroenterology 2009;136:1272–80.
13. Lok AS, Lai CL. Acute exacerbations in Chinese patients with chronic hepatitis B virus (HBV) infection. Incidence, predisposing factors and etiology. J Hepatol 1990;10:29–34.
14. Lai M, Hyatt BJ, Nasser I, et al. The clinical significance of persistently normal ALT in chronic hepatitis B infection. J Hepatol 2007;47:760–7.

15. Papatheodoridis GV, Manolakopoulos S, Liaw YF, et al. Follow-up and indications for liver biopsy in HBeAg-negative chronic hepatitis B virus infection with persistently normal ALT: a systematic review. J Hepatol 2012;57:196–202.

16. Kumar M, Sarin SK, Hissar S, et al. Virologic and histologic features of chronic hepatitis B virus-infected asymptomatic patients with persistently normal ALT. Gastroenterology 2008;134:1376–84.

17. Carman WF, Jacyna MR, Hadziyannis S, et al. Mutation preventing formation of hepatitis B e antigen in patients with chronic hepatitis B infection. Lancet 1989; 2:588–91.

18. Okamoto H, Tsuda F, Akahane Y, et al. Hepatitis B virus with mutations in the core promoter for an e antigen-negative phenotype in carriers with antibody to e antigen. J Virol 1994;68:8102–10.

19. Alward WL, McMahon BJ, Hall DB, et al. The long-term serological course of asymptomatic hepatitis B virus carriers and the development of primary hepatocellular carcinoma. J Infect Dis 1985;151:604–9.

20. Liu J, Yang HI, lee MH, et al. Incidence and determinants of spontaneous hepatitis B surface antigen seroclearance: a community-based follow-up study. Gastroenterology 2010;139:474–82.

21. Yuen MF, Wong DK, Sablon E, et al. HBsAg seroclearance in chronic hepatitis B in the Chinese: virological, histological, and clinical aspects. Hepatology 2004; 39:1694–701.

22. Huo TI, Wu JC, Lee PC, et al. Sero-clearance of hepatitis B surface antigen in chronic carriers does not necessarily imply a good prognosis. Hepatology 1998;28:231–6.

23. Yuen MF, Wong DK, Fung J, et al. HBsAg seroclearance in chronic hepatitis B in Asian patients: replicative level and risk of hepatocellular carcinoma. Gastroenterology 2008;135:1192–9.

24. Fattovich G, Bortolotti F, Donato F. Natural history of chronic hepatitis B: special emphasis on disease progression and prognostic factors. J Hepatol 2008;48: 335–52.

25. Chu CM, Liaw YF. Chronic hepatitis B virus infection acquired in childhood: special emphasis on prognostic and therapeutic implication of delayed HBeAg seroconversion. J Viral Hepat 2007;14:147–52.

26. Chu CM, Liaw YF. Predictive factors for reactivation of hepatitis B following hepatitis B e antigen seroconversion in chronic hepatitis B. Gastroenterology 2007; 133:1458–65.

27. Iloeje UH, Yang HI, Su J, et al. Predicting cirrhosis risk based on the level of circulating hepatitis B viral load. Gastroenterology 2006;130:678–86.

28. Chen CJ, Yang HI, Su J, et al. Risk of hepatocellular carcinoma across a biological gradient of serum hepatitis B virus DNA level. JAMA 2006;295:65–73.

29. Tseng TC, Liu CJ, Yang HC, et al. Serum hepatitis B surface antigen levels help predict disease progression in patients with low hepatitis B virus loads. Hepatology 2013;57:441–50.

30. Liaw YF. Role of hepatitis C virus in dual and triple hepatitis virus infection. Hepatology 1995;22:1101–8.

31. Pontisso P, Ruvoletto MG, Fattovich G, et al. Clinical and virological profiles in patients with multiple hepatitis virus infections. Gastroenterology 1993;105: 1529.

32. Sheen IS, Liaw YF, Lin DY, et al. Role of hepatitis C and delta viruses in the termination of chronic hepatitis B surface antigen carrier state: a multivariate analysis in a longitudinal follow-up study. J Infect Dis 1994;170:358–61.

33. Fong TL, Di Bisceglie AM, Waggoner JG, et al. The significance of antibody to hepatitis C virus in patients with chronic hepatitis B. Hepatology 1991;14:64–7.
34. Smedile A, Farci P, Verme G, et al. Influence of delta infection on severity of hepatitis B. Lancet 1982;2:945–7.
35. Pastore G, Monno L, Santantino T, et al. Hepatitis B virus clearance from serum and liver after acute hepatitis delta virus superinfection in chronic HBsAg carriers. J Med Virol 1990;31:284–90.
36. Fattovich G, Boscaro S, Noventa F, et al. Influence of hepatitis delta virus infection on progression to cirrhosis in chronic hepatitis type B. J Infect Dis 1987;155: 931–5.
37. Sagnelli E, Piccinino F, Pasquale G, et al. Delta agent infection: an unfavorable event in HBsAg positive chronic hepatitis. Liver 1984;4:170–6.
38. European Association For The Study Of The Liver. EASL clinical practice guidelines: management of chronic hepatitis B infection. J Hepatol 2012;57:167–85.
39. McQuillan GM, Coleman PJ, Kruszon-Moran D, et al. Prevalence of hepatitis B infection in the United States: the National Health and Nutrition Examination Surveys, 1976 through 1994. Am J Public Health 1999;89:14–8.
40. Kondo Y, Tsukada K, Takeuchi T, et al. High carrier rate after hepatitis B infection in the elderly. Hepatology 1993;18:768–74.
41. Yang HI, Lu SN, Liaw YF, et al. Hepatitis B e antigen and the risk of hepatocellular carcinoma. N Engl J Med 2002;347:168–74.
42. Sugauchi F, Mizokami M, Orito E, et al. Hepatitis B virus infection among residents of a nursing home for the elderly: seroepidemiological study and molecular evolutionary analysis. J Med Virol 2000;62:456–62.
43. Ghany E, Strader D, Thomas D, et al. Diagnosis, management and treatment of hepatitis C: an update. Hepatology 2009;49:1335–74.
44. Thein HH, Yi Q, Dore GJ, et al. Estimation of stage-specific fibrosis progression rates in chronic hepatitis C infection: a meta-analysis and meta-regression. Hepatology 2008;48:418–31.
45. Tong MJ, el-Farra NS, Reikes AR, et al. Clinical outcomes after transfusion-associated hepatitis C. N Engl J Med 1995;332:1463–6.
46. Takahashi M, Yamada G, Miyamoto R, et al. Natural course of chronic hepatitis C. Am J Gastroenterol 1993;88:240–3.
47. Fattovich G, Giustina G, Degos F, et al. Morbidity and mortality in compensated cirrhosis type C: a retrospective follow-up study of 384 patients. Gastroenterology 1997;112:463–72.
48. Bruno S, Crosignani A, Maisonneuve P, et al. Hepatitis C virus genotype 1b as a major risk factor associated with hepatocellular carcinoma in patients with cirrhosis: a seventeen year prospective cohort study. Hepatology 2007;46:1350–6.
49. Smith BD, Morgan RL, Beckett GA, et al. Recommendations for the identification of chronic hepatitis C virus infection among persons born during 1945–1965. MMWR Recomm Rep 2012;61:1–32.
50. Moyer VA, on behalf of the U.S. Preventative Services Task Force. Screening for hepatitis C virus infection in adults: US Preventive Services Task Force recommendation statement. Ann Intern Med 2013. http://dx.doi.org/10.7326/0003-4819-159-5-201309030-00672.
51. Cacoub P, Ratziu V, Myers RP, et al. Impact of treatment of extrahepatic manifestations in patients with chronic hepatitis C. J Hepatol 2002;36:812–8.
52. Piche T, Vanbiervliet G, Cherik F, et al. Effect of ondansetron, a 5-HT3 receptor antagonist, on fatigue in chronic hepatitis C: a randomized, double-blind, placebo controlled study. Gut 2005;54:1169–73.

53. Cacoub P, Renou C, Rosenthal E, et al. Extrahepatic manifestations associated with hepatitis C virus infection. A prospective multicenter study of 321 patients. The GERMIVIC. Groupe d'Etude et de Recherche en Medecine Interne et Maladies Infectieuses sur le Virus de l'Hepatitis C. Medicine (Baltimore) 2000;79: 47–56.

54. Swain MG, Lai MY, Shiffman ML, et al. A sustained virologic response is durable in patients with chronic hepatitis C treated with peginterferon alfa-2a and ribavirin. Gastroenterology 2010;139:1593–601.

55. Ng V, Saab S. Effects of a sustained virologic response on outcomes of patients with chronic hepatitis C. Clin Gastroenterol Hepatol 2011;9:923–30.

56. Backus L, Boothroyd DB, Phillips BR, et al. A sustained virologic response reduces risk of all cause mortality in patients with hepatitis C. Clin Gastroenterol Hepatol 2011;9:509–16.

57. Morgan RL, Baack B, Smith BD, et al. Eradication of hepatitis C virus infection and the development of hepatocellular carcinoma: a meta-analysis of observational studies. Ann Intern Med 2013;158:329–37.

58. Ziol M, Handra-Luca A, Kettaneh A, et al. Noninvasive assessment of liver fibrosis by measurement of stiffness in patients with chronic hepatitis C. Hepatology 2005;41:48–54.

59. Talwalkar JA, Kurtz DM, Schoenlever SJ, et al. Ultrasound-based transient elastography for the detection of hepatic fibrosis: systematic review and meta-analysis. Clin Gastroenterol Hepatol 2007;5:1214–20.

60. Ghany MG, Nelson D, Strader D, et al. An update on genotype 1 chronic hepatitis C viral infection: 2011 practice guidelines by the American Association for the Study of Liver Diseases. Hepatology 2011;54:1433–44.

61. Chou R, Hartung D, Rahman B, et al. Comparative effectiveness of antiviral treatment for hepatitis C virus infection in adults: a systematic review. Ann Intern Med 2013;158:114–23.

62. Lawitz E, Lalezari JP, Hassanein T, et al. Sofosbuvir in combination with peginterferon alfa-2a and ribavirin for non-cirrhotic, treatment naïve patients with genotypes 1, 2 and 3 hepatitis C infection: a randomized, double blind, phase 2 trial. Lancet Infect Dis 2013;13:401–8.

63. Kowdley KV, Lawitz E, Crespo I, et al. Sofosbuvir with pegylated interferon alfa 2a and ribavirin for treatment-naïve patients with hepatitis C genoypte-1 infection (ATOMIC): an open-label, randomized, multicenter phase 2 trial. Lancet 2013;381:2100–7.

64. Gane EJ, Stedman CA, Hyland RH, et al. Nucleotide polymerase inhibitor sofosbuvir plus ribavirin for hepatitis C. N Engl J Med 2013;368:34.

65. Lawitz E, Mangia A, Wyles D, et al. Sofosbuvir for previously untreated chronic hepatitis C infection. N Engl J Med 2013;368:1878–87.

66. World Health Organization. Hepatitis C. Available at: http://www.who.int/mediacentre/factsheets/fs164/en/. Accessed August 25, 2013.

67. Cainelli F. Hepatitis C virus infection in the elderly: epidemiology, natural history and management. Drugs Aging 2008;25:9–18.

68. Alter MJ, Kruszon-Moran D, Nainan OV. The prevalence of hepatitis C virus infection in the United States 1988-1994. N Engl J Med 1999;341:556–62.

69. Armstrong GL, Wasley A, Simard EP, et al. The prevalence of hepatitis C virus infection in the United States 1999-2002. Ann Intern Med 2006;144:705–14.

70. Baldo V, Floreani A, Menegon T. Prevalence of antibodies against hepatitis C in the elderly: a seroepidemiological study in a nursing home and in an open population. Gerontology 2000;46:194–8.

71. Monica F, Lirussi F, Nassuato G. Hepatitis C virus infection and related chronic liver disease in a resident elderly population: the Silea study. J Viral Hepat 1998; 5:345–51.

72. Sawabe M, Arai T, Esaki Y. Persistent infection of hepatitis C virus in the elderly. Q J Med 1996;89:291–6.

73. Thabut D, Le Calvez S, Thibault V, et al. Hepatitis C in 6865 patients 65 years old or older: a severe and neglected curable disease? Am J Gastroenterol 2006; 101:1260–7.

74. Minola E, Prati D, Suter F, et al. Age at infection affects the long term outcome of transfusion associated chronic hepatitis C. Blood 2002;99:4588–91.

75. Monica F, Lirussi F, Pregan I, et al. Hepatitis C infection in a resident elderly population: a 10 year follow up study. Dig Liver Dis 2006;38:336–40.

76. Ohishi W, Kitamoto M, Aikata H. Impact of aging on the development of hepatocellular carcinoma in patients with hepatitis C infection in Japan. Scand J Gastroenterol 2003;38:894–900.

77. NIH consensus conference on management of hepatitis C 2002. NIH Consens State Sci Statements 2002;19:1–46.

78. Floreani A, Minola E, Carden I, et al. Are elderly patients poor candidates for pegylated interferon and ribavirin therapy in the treatment of chronic hepatitis C. J Am Geriatr Soc 2006;54:549–50.

Index

Note: Page numbers of article titles are in **boldface** type.

Clin Geriatr Med 30 (2014) 169–174
http://dx.doi.org/10.1016/S0749-0690(13)00103-1
0749-0690/14/$ – see front matter © 2014 Elsevier Inc. All rights reserved.

geriatric.theclinics.com

Moving?

Make sure your subscription moves with you!

To notify us of your new address, find your **Clinics Account Number** (located on your mailing label above your name), and contact customer service at:

Email: journalscustomerservice-usa@elsevier.com

800-654-2452 (subscribers in the U.S. & Canada)
314-447-8871 (subscribers outside of the U.S. & Canada)

Fax number: 314-447-8029

Elsevier Health Sciences Division
Subscription Customer Service
3251 Riverport Lane
Maryland Heights, MO 63043

*To ensure uninterrupted delivery of your subscription, please notify us at least 4 weeks in advance of move.

Printed and bound by CPI Group (UK) Ltd, Croydon, CR0 4YY

03/10/2024

01040497-0017